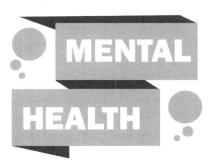

MENTAL
HEALTH

A WHOLE SCHOOL APPROACH

POSITIVE MENTAL HEALTH

This new series of texts presents a modern and comprehensive set of evidence-based strategies for promoting positive mental health in schools. There is a growing prevalence of mental ill health among children and young people within a context of funding cuts, strained services and a lack of formal training for teachers. The series recognises the complexity of the issues involved, the vital role that teachers play, and the current education and health policy frameworks in order to provide practical guidance backed up by the latest research.

ACKNOWLEDGMENTS

Grateful thanks to:

Noelle Doona

Keith Ellis

Chris Goodall

Corinne Latham

Our titles are also available in a range of electronic formats. To order, or for details of our bulk discounts, please go to our website www. criticalpublishing.com or contact our distributor, NBN International, 10 Thornbury Road, Plymouth PL6 7PP, telephone 01752 202301 or email orders@nbninternational.com.

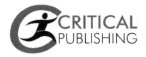

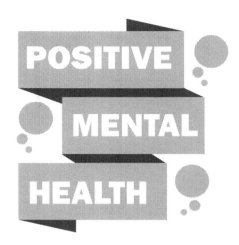

A WHOLE SCHOOL APPROACH

Jonathan Glazzard and Rachel Bostwick

First published in 2018 by Critical Publishing Ltd

British Library Cataloguing in Publication Data
A CIP record for this book is available from the British Library

ISBN: 978-1-912096-08-4

This book is also available in the following e-book formats:

MOBI ISBN: 978-1-912096-07-7
EPUB ISBN: 978-1-912096-06-0
Adobe e-book ISBN: 978-1-912096-05-3

Cover and text design by Out of House Limited
Project Management by Out of House Publishing Solutions
Printed and bound in Great Britain by 4edge, Essex

Critical Publishing
3 Connaught Road
St Albans
AL3 5RX

www.criticalpublishing.com

Paper from responsible sources

+CONTENTS

+ MEET THE SERIES EDITOR AND AUTHORS

JONATHAN GLAZZARD

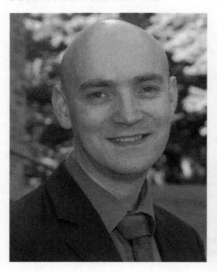

RACHEL BOSTWICK

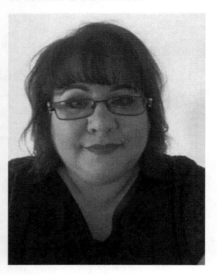

Jonathan Glazzard is series editor for *Positive Mental Health*. He is Professor of Teacher Education at Leeds Beckett University and also the professor attached to the Carnegie Centre of Excellence for Mental Health in Schools. He teaches across a range of QTS and non-QTS programmes and is an experienced teacher educator.

Rachel Bostwick is Senior Partnership and Enterprise Consultant and leads the Carnegie Centre of Excellence for Mental Health in Schools and the School Mental Health Award, which exists to strengthen the mental health of the next generation by supporting schools to make a positive change at all levels.

✚ INTRODUCTION

This book supports teachers and school leaders to develop a whole school approach to mental health. Mental health is not the same thing as mental illness. Everyone has mental health and there is a need to de-stigmatise the term. It is important for teachers and school leaders to create a school culture which enables everyone who is part of the school community to talk openly about mental health.

As a teacher or school leader you are responsible for, or will contribute to, creating a school culture which promotes positive mental health. Creating a sense of belonging for all members of the school community is important. This will help to promote well-being. Developing a curriculum which explicitly teaches children about mental health is vital for developing students' mental health literacy. Creating systems for identifying mental health needs will ensure that students do not slip through the net.

We know that one in ten children currently has some form of diagnosable mental health need (DfE, 2016). Young people are exposed to multiple influences and risk factors which can have detrimental impacts on their mental health, and some children are more vulnerable than others. The pressures on young people appear to be increasing. They are subjected to a challenging academic curriculum and high-stakes testing from a young age. The links between social media and mental health are also now documented. The links been poverty and mental health are well established. However, the causes will vary across individuals and the solutions need to be personalised to individuals rather than generic.

This book has been written at a time when the government is investing in mental health. The Green Paper, published in December 2017, identifies a bold set of proposals to address children and young people's mental health including the introduction of Designated Senior Leaders of Mental Health in schools and access for schools to Mental Health Support Teams. Currently, waiting lists to access specialist services are too long and too many young people do not meet the threshold criteria for referral. Consequently, support often comes too late or not at all. The responsibility is often placed on schools to address pupils' mental health needs, yet teachers feel inadequately prepared to undertake this task.

This book supports you to develop your mental health provision. However, new challenges will continue to emerge to which schools will need to respond. At the time of completing this book, gaming disorder has been identified as a new mental health need. This illustrates the need for teachers to continually update their knowledge and the need for high-quality professional development to enable them to do this.

It is important to avoid stereotypes. Children and young people who are born into social deprivation will not inevitably develop a mental health need. Children from high-income families do develop mental health needs. While some groups of young people are more vulnerable than others, not all children who are living in care have mental health needs. Children who are polite, high performing, well behaved and dressed smartly may have mental health needs but these may be invisible. Young people may appear to be coping well but may be hiding serious mental health needs. Systems of identification in schools need to catch all these children.

This book provides a concise text for busy teachers and school leaders detailing what you need to know to help inform your school's approach to mental health. It contains a number of features that highlight particular types of information. Research boxes are indicated by a magnifying glass symbol and statistics boxes have a bar graph icon. There are also professional links, case studies and critical questions along with helpful objectives, checklists and summaries.

We hope that you find this book useful and informative.

Jonathan Glazzard and Rachel Bostwick

✚ CHAPTER 1

WHAT IS MENTAL HEALTH?

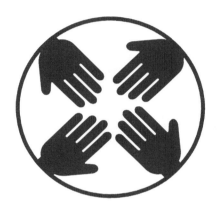

PROFESSIONAL LINKS

This chapter addresses the following:

- *Keeping Children Safe in Education: Statutory Guidance for Schools and Colleges* (DfE, 2016).
- The Equality Act 2010.
- The *Special Educational Needs and Disability Code of Practice: 0 to 25 Years* (DfE, 2015).

CHAPTER OBJECTIVES

By the end of this chapter you will understand:

+ what mental health is;

+ your legal responsibilities in relation to supporting children and young people with mental health needs;

+ types of mental health needs;

+ the role of schools in promoting positive mental health in children and young people.

INTRODUCTION

This chapter outlines what we mean by mental health and provides an overview of the contribution that primary and secondary schools can make to the promotion of good mental health. Evidence suggests that mental health needs appear to be increasing (Burton, 2014). One in ten children has a diagnosable mental health condition (DfE/DH, 2017), and girls are particularly at risk of developing a low sense of well-being (Danby and Hamilton, 2016). While this is concerning, it is also possible that increased public awareness of mental health has resulted in more effective identification and diagnosis processes (Burton, 2014).

Research demonstrates that there are multiple risk factors which result in mental health needs. These include: income inequality; relationship breakdown; parental conflict; parental health; school expectations; bullying, including digital bullying and concerns about body image (Bor et al, 2014; Danby and Hamilton, 2016). Other risk factors include low self-esteem, abuse, neglect, socio-economic disadvantage, peer influences and grief or loss (DfE, 2016).

Research demonstrates that an increasing number of children and young people are demonstrating self-harm, phobia, depression, anxiety, substance misuse, attachment disorders, conduct disorders and eating disorders (DfE, 2014; Dickins, 2014; Sisak et al, 2014). There is evidence to suggest that children and young people with special educational needs are more at risk of developing mental health conditions (Lindsay and Dockrell, 2012) and those exposed to multiple risk factors demonstrate a significantly increased risk (Weare, 2010).

Children and young people with mental health needs are at risk of being absent from school and underachieving academically (DH, 2014). While schools can have a positive impact by developing universal approaches for all pupils and addressing the specific needs of those who require targeted support, it has been emphasised that schools cannot meet the mental health needs of all pupils in isolation (O'Hara, 2014). Some pupils will require specialist provision, particularly in cases where needs are complex and where there is risk of harm to the child.

WHAT IS MENTAL HEALTH?

The following perspective has been adopted by the World Health Organisation:

Health is a state of complete physical, mental and social well-being and not merely the absence of disease or infirmity... Mental health is defined as a state of well-being in which every individual realizes his or her own potential, can cope with the normal stresses of life, can work productively and fruitfully, and is able to make a contribution to her or his community.

(WHO, 2014)

Contemporary perspectives on health position mental health as a positive concept rather than as a deficit attribute within a person (Weare, 2010; Weare and Markham, 2005). Thus, mental health has been conceptualised as a continuum, with good mental health at one end of the spectrum and mental illness at the other end (Danby and Hamilton, 2016). It is critical that children and young people understand that everyone has mental health and that this lies somewhere along this continuum; there will be times when most people need more support than at other times (Prever, 2006) and being able to recognise this is crucial in order to make positive changes. Thus, helping young people to understand firstly, that mental health exists within a state of flux and secondly, that they can largely control it, can provide them with a sense of agency. Mental health moves along a continuum and is influenced by a range of social, biological and psychological factors. Helping children to understand what factors they can change and what individual and external resources they can draw on for support are important ways of empowering young people to take greater responsibility for their own mental health.

The physical, social, psychological and emotional aspects of health overlap and interrelate (Danby and Hamilton, 2016). Children and young people's mental health is influenced by the quality of relationships they form with peers and adults (Thapa et al, 2013). This is known as social connectedness (Aldridge and Chesney, 2018). Engagement in physical activity can also improve mental health. However, while social connections and physical activity can improve mental health, having good mental health can also impact on the extent to which young people choose to participate in establishing social connections and physical activity.

Tabloid coverage can result in negative assumptions and stigma (Barber, 2012) in relation to mental health. This can lead to practitioners and parents forming a deficit view which associates mental health with mental illness (Holstrom, 2013; Time to Change, 2015). Schools play an important role in reducing stigma by helping children to understand that mental health is a fundamental aspect of everyone's health. By mainstreaming conversations about mental health, schools can help young people to understand that mental health is not something to be ashamed of. The stigmatisation of mental health can have detrimental effects (Danby and Hamilton, 2016) because it can reduce the willingness of individuals to talk about their needs.

School leaders and teachers have a responsibility for providing safe, caring and nurturing environments so that all pupils can thrive. However, it has been argued that there is a danger of viewing young children as psychologically and emotionally vulnerable (Ecclestone, 2014, 2015), particularly when they display specific reactions to daily experiences which influence their emotions. Schools therefore play an important role in promoting young people's resilience to adverse situations so that they can 'bounce back' from these.

Certain risk factors are linked to mental health needs. These include:

+ *parental conflict;*

+ *income inequality;*

+ *parental relationship breakdown;*

+ *parental health;*

+ *cyberbullying;*

+ *school expectations;*

+ *special educational needs/additional learning needs;*

+ *school environment.*

(Danby and Hamilton, 2016)

CRITICAL QUESTIONS

+ Some life experiences are more challenging than others and will demand greater resilience to respond to them. What experiences might these include?

+ What contributions can role models make to reducing stigma about mental health?

+ What factors can protect against young people developing mental health needs?

LEGAL RESPONSIBILITIES

The following legislation or guidance places a duty on schools to safeguard and promote the welfare of children and young people:

+ Section 175 of the Education Act 2002 duty applies to maintained schools.

+ The Education (Independent School Standards) Regulations 2014 applies to independent schools (which include free schools and academies).

+ The Non-Maintained Special Schools (England) Regulations 2015 place a duty on non-maintained special schools to promote the welfare of children and young people.

+ The Sexual Offences Act 2003 states that it is an offence for a person aged 18 or over (eg teacher, youth worker) to have a sexual relationship with a child under 18 where that person is in a position of trust in respect of that child, even if the relationship is consensual.

+ All schools must have regard to the following document: *Keeping Children Safe in Education: Statutory Guidance for Schools and Colleges* (DfE, 2016).

+ The Equality Act 2010: schools must prevent direct or indirect discrimination of individuals with protected characteristics. Disability is one protected characteristic, and this includes mental health conditions. This legislation places a duty on schools to provide reasonable adjustments to ensure equality of opportunity for individuals with protected characteristics. It is important to remember the multi-sectional nature of protected characteristics and thus, individuals may have one or more of these.

+ The *Special Educational Needs and Disability Code of Practice: 0 to 25 Years* (DfE, 2015): mental health is now recognised for the first time as a special educational need and schools have a duty to work in partnership with pupils, parents and external agencies to support pupils' mental health needs. The code emphasises the importance of early identification and intervention for all those with identified special educational needs and disabilities.

CRITICAL QUESTIONS

To meet these duties how might schools:

+ create a culture which promote a sense of belonging?

+ develop approaches to support the identification of mental health needs?

+ develop the curriculum so that mental health is a taught aspect of it?

+ develop policies on teaching, learning, assessment and behaviour management which reduce the risk of mental health needs occurring?

+ develop approaches for working with parents, carers and external agencies to ensure that the needs of the child are met?

+ develop approaches to monitoring the impact of interventions?

+ develop mechanisms for providing children and young people with mental health needs with a voice so that they can participate in decision-making?

+ develop approaches to professional development in mental health for all staff?

MENTAL HEALTH AND ACADEMIC ATTAINMENT

Research indicates that well-planned and well-implemented opportunities for supporting the well-being of students can positively affect academic outcomes (Greenberg et al, 2003; Gumora and Arsenio, 2002; Malecki and Elliott, 2002; Teo et al, 1996; Welsh et al, 2001; Wentzel,

1993; Wood, 2006; Zins et al, 2004). According to Sammons (2007), there are strong relationships between student behaviour, attainment and learning and their social and emotional development. Due to the relationships between mental health, academic success and life oppor-tunities, schools have a critical role to play in promoting students' mental well-being (Clausson and Berg, 2008; Cushman et al, 2011).

CRITICAL QUESTIONS

+ Do you agree that schools have an important role to play in promoting students' well-being? Explain your answer to this.
+ Should schools prioritise students' academic development or their well-being?

MENTAL HEALTH IN PRIMARY SCHOOLS

The following section outlines the common needs which you may notice in primary schools. There are other needs that are mentioned later in this chapter which may occur in primary schools but more commonly occur during adolescence.

CONDUCT DISORDERS

Children with conduct disorders may demonstrate verbal and physical aggression, defiance and anti-social behaviour. They may need support to understand what is meant by socially accepted behaviour and the impact of their behaviour on others. Approaches used in schools to support children with conduct disorders may reflect a behaviourist approach which emphasises the use of rewards and sanctions. Some children may require a highly individual rewards and sanctions system which differs from the system used for all pupils. Behaviourist approaches focus on the consequences of behaviour rather than the causes. In contrast, an alternative approach stems from a branch of psychology known as humanism. Humanism attempts to focus on developing the child's sense of self through improving their self-concept and self-esteem. It focuses on helping the child to recognise their strengths and is underpinned by the work of Maslow and Rogers who argued that a positive sense of self is essential to enable an individual to achieve their full potential.

ANXIETY

Anxiety disorders range in type and severity. Anxiety may be related to a specific phobia, for example a fear of an object, or situation. Children may become anxious in unfamiliar situations and may be anxious in some situations but not in others. Some children may be anxious all the time. In addition, anxiety might result from separation from a significant other. Children with anxiety may display a range of symptoms. These include fearfulness, irritability, panic, breathlessness and sleep deprivation (DfE, 2016).

ATTACHMENT DISORDERS

The work of Bowlby helped to demonstrate the significance of positive attachments between children and their primary caregivers. In cases where loving, caring and secure attachments are not formed because of the family context, this can have a detrimental impact on the child's sense of self and their behaviour. Children with attachment disorders may be withdrawn, demonstrate anti-social behaviour, have low confidence and a negative perception of their abilities. Forming positive and secure relationships with children is essential, particularly in cases where attachments with their primary caregivers are weak, non-existent or absent. Some children with attachment disorders may benefit from interventions which help them to develop a positive sense of self.

CRITICAL QUESTIONS

+ What situations in school may result in a child feeling anxious?

+ What are the advantages and disadvantages of supporting conduct disorders through a behaviourist approach?

+ What are the advantages and disadvantages of supporting conduct disorders through a solution-focused approach which involves the child in setting goals and supports them in recognising their own strengths?

CASE STUDY

One primary school decided to introduce a universal approach to supporting children's well-being. Rather than focusing only on children who presented needs, they used the resources from the Head Start resources with all children. They selected resources from the toolkit: www.corc.uk.net/media/1506/primary-school-measures_310317_forweb.pdf.

They decided to adopt the feelings survey and the resilience survey, which all children completed once a term. This allowed teachers to identify any children with specific needs and provide appropriate support, but it also enabled senior leaders to identify differences in feelings and resilience between specific groups of children (for example, gender, ethnicity, age and special educational needs).

● Nearly 8 per cent of children aged 5–10 have a diagnosable mental health need.

● Mental health needs are more common in boys (just over 11 per cent) than girls (nearly 8 per cent).

● Around 1 in 10 white children have a mental health disorder, compared to just under 1 in 10 black children, and 3 in 100 Indian children.

(DfE, 2016)

CRITICAL QUESTION

+ Why do you think there are variations in the statistics in relation to gender and ethnicity?

Research by Danby and Hamilton (2016) found that primary practitioners tended to focus on developing children's understanding of feelings and promoting their resilience. However, they were reluctant to use the term 'mental health' with children as they perceived this to be an unsuitable term to use with children. This can result in children forming negative conceptions about mental health, which can result in stigma. The danger is that these attitudes can make discussions about mental health awkward and it becomes taboo.

CRITICAL QUESTIONS

+ What are your views on the use of the term 'mental health' with young children?

+ What are the benefits of using the term 'mental health' with young children?

+ What issues may result from using the term 'mental health' with young children?

+ How might you overcome these issues?

MENTAL HEALTH IN SECONDARY SCHOOLS

This section addresses common mental health needs in secondary schools. Needs that have been identified earlier in this chapter may also be evident in secondary schools. Specific mental health needs may also co-exist alongside other mental health needs or may exist alongside other identified needs.

DEPRESSION

Depression exists along a spectrum which ranges from mild to severe. It can fluctuate depending on personal experiences and can affect a child's ability to learn. Children may become withdrawn, tearful, and demonstrate persistent low mood. They may demonstrate decreased energy, sleeplessness and loss of appetite. Engagement in physical activity, social activity and a healthy diet can alleviate depression. Supporting a young person to experience success can also help. It is important to encourage young people to talk about how they feel and for responsible adults to become good listeners. You will need to demonstrate patience and empathy.

SELF-HARM

Self-harm can include hitting, cutting, burning, picking skin, pulling hair, over-dosing and self-strangulation. It is particularly worrying that children can now access websites which promote self-harm and normalise it, and it is also a concern that the process of self-harm can now be viewed through live streaming on the internet. Self-harm may co-exist alongside other conditions such as stress, anxiety and depression, and it might be a response to these conditions. It may also be a response to abuse, neglect and other traumatic incidents.

The personal, social and emotional (PSE) curriculum should introduce children to the dangers of self-harm at an age-appropriate level. You will need to be observant in identifying self-harm and if you suspect self-harm then you have a responsibility to report this to the designated person in school. They should guide you on the next steps and provide advice about how to raise your concerns with parents.

EATING DISORDERS

Eating disorders include anorexia nervosa and bulimia nervosa. Both disorders are associated with a desire to be thin and body image concerns. Signs could include sudden loss of appetite, loss of weight, vomiting after food, anxiety or depression. Children with eating disorders may require specialist support from the health profession.

Children's body image may be negatively influenced by advertising and the media (including social media) and peer influences. Research indicates that advertisements often portray idealised images of beauty (Frith, 2017), which impacts negatively on body confidence. Females are often depicted through images of slender bodies which are used to represent beauty and perfection (Frith, 2017). Images and messages about 'perfect' bodies are internalised, and this can lead to children and young people making unrealistic comparisons between the media images and their own bodies. This can result in low body esteem.

While the research suggests that females may be more prone to poor body image than males, boys and young men can also be affected (British Youth Council, 2017). Advertisements which portray the perfect male body often depict muscular strength as a characteristic of the ideal male body. Research suggests that this can result in males developing an obsession with muscle building, as a result developing body dissatisfaction (British Youth Council, 2017).

Schools need to address the theme of body image through the PSE curriculum. Children should be supported to challenge the stereotypes that they are exposed to in the media. Additionally, the science curriculum will introduce children to the importance of a healthy balanced diet. If you suspect that a child may have developed an eating disorder, this needs to be addressed sensitively. Talk to the person with responsibility for mental health in the school and discuss how to raise your concerns with the child's parent(s) or carer(s).

CRITICAL QUESTIONS

+ What contribution might the examination system in secondary schools make to students' mental health needs?
+ Why might adolescence be a particularly vulnerable time for young people?
+ How might peer pressure influence mental health during adolescence?
+ How might social media influence mental health during adolescence?

CASE STUDY

A secondary school decided to use the Warwick-Edinburgh Mental Well-being Scale, the perceived stress scale and the student resilience survey from the Head Start resources: www.corc.uk.net/media/1506/primary-school-measures_310317_forweb.pdf.

The stress scale was used with all students in Years 10 and 11 while they were undertaking their GCSE courses. The students completed it once a term. The other two surveys were completed by all students at the start of each academic year. The perceived stress scale was particularly useful as it allowed teachers to identify students who felt they were experiencing stress. The pastoral leader then met with these students to discuss the factors that had contributed to them feeling stressed. Strategies were established by the school to support these students at a critical time in their academic development. Students were asked to make suggestions of strategies which they felt would help them, and the pastoral leader also suggested strategies for alleviating stress. One of the outcomes was the introduction of a dedicated room for students to use for revision purposes in preparation for the examinations. This was particularly useful for students who did not have adequate revision space at home. Some students were given planners to help them organise their workload, and all students who perceived they were experiencing stress were provided with lessons on stress management. This included mindfulness activities and physical activity sessions during the school day.

- In 2014, 18 per cent of young people aged 11–15 reported they had experienced some form of cyberbullying.

- 12 per cent of those aged 11–15 reported that they had a mental health need.

- There has been a 68 per cent increase in self-harm rates among girls aged 13 to 16 since 2011.

- 45 per cent of looked after children have a diagnosable mental disorder (compared to 10 per cent of all children).

(DfE, 2016)

Research indicates that an engaging environment that supports the active participation of young people in the school plays a protective role in relation to physical, social and emotional health, and enables young people to thrive academically (Butcher, 2010; Noble and Toft, 2010). Central to such thinking is the concept of school 'connectedness'. This is where students believe that adults in the school care about them as individuals and care about their learning (Blum and Libbey, 2004). Greater school connectedness reduces the likelihood that young people will engage in health-compromising behaviours and increases the likelihood of academic success (Klem and Connell, 2004). Research has also shown that young people who report high levels of school connectedness report lower levels of emotional distress and risk-taking behaviours (Blum and Libbey, 2004). Research has shown that students who lack social and emotional skills often become less connected to school as they get older. This lack of connection has been found to have a negative impact on their academic attainment, behaviour and health (Durlak et al, 2011). Students with low school connectedness are two to three times more likely to experience mental health symptoms compared to more connected peers (Glover et al, 1998).

SUMMARY

Teachers are not mental health experts. However, there is much that schools can do to promote positive mental health. Fundamental to this is the role of school culture in establishing a climate where students feel that they belong. The role of teachers and other practitioners in establishing positive relationships with students is critical to establishing school connectedness. It appears that the prevalence of mental health needs among children and young people is increasing. However, mental health should no longer be seen as a stigma; it is something that everyone has, and it is not synonymous with mental illness. Young people are subjected to the influences of the societies in which they live. Their mental health is influenced by a range of complex social, environmental, cultural and political factors which are not always positive. There are no quick fixes, but we can start by supporting young people to understand what mental health is and we can provide them with some tools to help them develop positive well-being. Schools play a vital role in relation to both identification of needs and intervention. Mental health and academic achievement are inter-related and the most effective schools place student well-being at the heart of any school improvement plan.

CHECKLIST

This chapter has addressed:

✓ what is meant by mental health;

✓ the role of schools in promoting a positive culture;

✓ key mental health needs;

✓ ways in which schools might assess young people's well-being.

FURTHER READING

Adelman, H S and Taylor, L (2015) *Mental Health in Schools: Engaging Learners, Preventing Problems, and Improving Schools*. New York: Skyhorse Publishing.

Holt, M K and Grills, A E (2015) *Critical Issues in School-based Mental Health: Evidence-based Research, Practice, and Interventions*. New York: Routledge.

+ **CHAPTER 2**

PROMOTING A WHOLE SCHOOL APPROACH TO POSITIVE MENTAL HEALTH

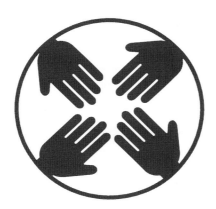

PROFESSIONAL LINKS

This chapter addresses the following:

Teachers must establish a safe and stimulating environment for pupils, rooted in mutual respect (TS1; DfE, 2011).

Teachers must have proper and professional regard for the ethos, policies and practices of the school in which they teach (TS, Part 2; DfE, 2011).

Special Educational Needs and Disability Code of Practice (DfE, 2015).

CHAPTER OBJECTIVES

After reading this chapter you will understand:

+ what a whole school approach to mental health looks like;
+ the importance of school culture and leadership;
+ the importance of taking care of staff mental health;
+ how to implement a whole school approach to mental health.

INTRODUCTION

In 2017 the Prime Minister was determined to correct, in her words, the 'historic injustice' of unfair discrimination and poor treatment of people with mental health needs. One in ten, or 850,000 children and young people, have a diagnosable mental health disorder. This chapter addresses whole school approaches to positive mental health.

Teachers are not health professionals. The key role of a teacher is to educate children and young people. They are not trained to diagnose mental health difficulties or to deliver psychological interventions. However, they spend much more time working with young people than professionals from health or social care services. There is a great deal that they can do to establish positive mental health in children and young people.

Addressing the problems experienced by young people is not sufficient. To promote a whole school approach to mental health, school leaders also have a responsibility to promote a positive sense of well-being for all staff. Teachers feel that poor teacher mental health affects detrimentally the quality of their teaching, pupils' learning and the quality of the relationships that teachers establish with pupils and colleagues (Glazzard, 2018).

Mental health operates along a continuum and it is important to distinguish between someone who is experiencing a mental health issue, such as stress or anxiety, and the diagnosis of a mental health issue. Some mental health issues are temporary or triggered by certain factors, and many people experience stress and anxiety. Others have greater permanency. Reducing the triggers will help to alleviate problems. In cases where problems are more persistent, teachers should be alert to the signs, which may indicate the need for referral and/or targeted interventions.

This chapter addresses ways in which schools can promote a whole school approach to mental health. We consider the role of the school culture, the policies of the school and the curriculum in engendering positive mental health for children, young people and adults who work in schools.

PROMOTING A POSITIVE SCHOOL CULTURE

Key to the development of a positive school culture is the creation of a whole-school vision. The vision should be underpinned by a set of values which demonstrate the school's commitment to challenging all forms of discrimination. The school's commitment to respect and equality of opportunity for all, collaboration, democracy and its commitment to diversity should be clearly visible. Through the vision and values statements schools can also demonstrate a commitment to safeguarding everyone who belongs to the school community. In addition, trust, loyalty, kindness and honesty are important character traits to emphasise within the values of a school. Senior leaders should develop approaches to involve all stakeholders in the development of the school vision and values statements to demonstrate a commitment to the principle of democracy.

It is essential that the vision and values are borne out in practice as well as being articulated within documentation. They apply to children, young people and adults, and therefore all members of the school community have a responsibility to uphold these. It is important for all members of that community to consider the effect of their words (written or verbal) and actions on other people and to ensure that everyone is treated with dignity and respect. Differences between individuals should be viewed as positive and there should be a climate of mutual trust and respect. School cultures which promote divisions between people, fear and secrecy are not positive places in which to work and learn.

All schools should promote a culture of listening that promotes openness on mental health issues rather than making them taboo. Schools should provide talks about mental health and additional support should be available, particularly at times when students may experience stress and anxiety, such as during examination periods. While students should be encouraged to do well in examinations, school leaders should ensure that this does not perpetuate mental health issues. Access to counselling and pastoral support in schools is critical in supporting students and staff with specific needs. Senior leaders should monitor systematically the impact of these approaches on outcomes for those who access these services. Additionally, leaders should monitor the impact of the anti-bullying policy and approaches to peer mentoring on outcomes for students.

Schools are beginning to monitor more systematically students' mental health and well-being in a similar way to the monitoring of student attainment. Regular assessments of all students' well-being using published well-being surveys is one way of doing this. This can support schools in identifying trends over time. Some schools have purchased sophisticated software packages, which provide teachers with well-being profiles of individual students as well as over-arching data for senior leaders who need to see variations by gender, ethnicity, special educational needs and/or disabilities, those students in receipt of pupil premium or other vulnerable students.

THE LEADERSHIP OF MENTAL HEALTH IN SCHOOLS

The Green Paper, *Transforming Children and Young People's Mental Health Provision* (DfE, 2017), recommends that a designated senior leader who is responsible for mental health should be available in every school. This appointment represents a strategic commitment to mental health and provides children, young people, staff, parents and external agencies with a point of contact. The senior leader can ensure that mental health provision is appropriately led, managed and evaluated across the school. A key part of the role is to focus on establishing whole school approaches which will promote good mental health in children and young people.

PROMOTING POSITIVE TEACHER MENTAL HEALTH

Research demonstrates that there are high levels of anxiety and stress-related health problems among teachers (Jeffcoat and Hayes, 2012) and that burnout and retention issues (Watson, 2014) are evident.

According to Dodge et al (2012), several factors influence teacher well-being. These include:

+ *their socio-economic status or financial security;*

+ *their sense of professional autonomy;*

+ *their sense of connectedness to other people and the school;*

+ *their sense of agency;*

+ *their beliefs about their personal competence.*

(Dodge et al, 2012)

The Education Support Partnership has identified some key factors which contribute to teacher well-being. These include:

+ *the demands of the job such as workload and work environment;*

+ *how much control they have, ie a person's own influence over how their job is carried out;*

+ *the level of support they receive from colleagues, their line-manager and the organisation;*

+ *the quality of relationships with colleagues and students to reduce conflict and deal with unacceptable behaviour;*

+ *their understanding of their role, ie their understanding of the job content and expectations;*

+ *the management of change, ie how change is managed in the organisation.*

(Education Support Partnership, 2017)

To enhance teacher well-being, school leaders should foster a climate which promotes trust and openness within collegiate relationships (Paterson and Grantham, 2016). Often, *'a problem shared is a problem halved'* (Paterson and Grantham, 2016) and it is critical that teachers can acknowledge both their strengths and weaknesses without fear of judgement. Research suggests that having their strengths recognised by the leadership team (Roffey, 2012) is critical to a positive sense of well-being, and teachers who are happy in their role will pass on a positive vibe to their pupils. Happy teachers produce happy pupils (Roffey, 2012).

Research suggests that video-enhanced reflective practice has been highlighted as a tool for providing positive feedback and developing skills that increase self-esteem and confidence (Strathie et al, 2011). This provides an opportunity for teachers to reflect on the strengths and weaknesses of their own teaching within a non-judgemental environment.

Senior leaders who support teachers to become better teachers, while also recognising their strengths and valuing them, engender a positive school culture which recognises that everyone has strengths and areas for development. Practising authentic leadership, where school leaders openly acknowledge their own strengths and weaknesses, promotes a healthy school culture.

Reducing excessive and unnecessary teacher workload is essential in promoting positive teacher well-being. The Department for Education (DfE) produced guidelines for school leaders in 2017 to support schools in reducing teacher workload. Among the key recommendations it was suggested that:

+ *all marking should be meaningful, manageable and motivating;*

+ *schools should spend time planning collaboratively, and engage with a professional body of knowledge and quality-assured resources;*

+ *in relation to data management, only collect what is needed to support outcomes for children. The amount of data collected should be proportionate to its usefulness.*

_____

(DfE, 2017)

However, addressing teacher workload will only solve part of the problem. In some schools, teachers perform their duties within a climate of fear. They may be subjected to excessive monitoring and surveillance through lesson observations, learning walks and scrutiny of planning and pupils' work. They may have been subjected to unrealistic expectations in relation to the progress of their students, including the assumption that all children should make progress in every lesson. This assumption is one which is unachievable and senior leaders who promote positive school cultures tend to adopt a broader perspective by evaluating progress over several weeks rather than in a single lesson. In some schools, cultures of surveillance operate everywhere. Surveillance is not only performed by senior leaders but circulates among all staff who hold various positions of power. Building cultures of collaboration and respect for all rather than cultures of surveillance is critical for positive well-being.

TEACHER WELL-BEING

The Education Support Partnership published research in 2017 which indicated that:

- 75 per cent of 1,250 school and college staff and leaders had experienced psychological, physical or behavioural symptoms because of their work.
- Additionally, 19 per cent reported that they had experienced panic attacks.
- 56 per cent had suffered from insomnia.
- 41 per cent had experienced difficulties concentrating.
- 52 per cent had been off for more than a month during the academic year.

EMBEDDING MENTAL HEALTH WITHIN SCHOOL POLICIES

School policies should be written with consideration given to how they might affect the mental health of children, young people or staff. Policies relating to planning, assessment and feedback, and data management should consider the latest guidance from the government on reducing teacher workload (DfE, 2017). Policies related to learning and teaching should take account of the impact of specific pedagogical approaches on pupils' mental health. Curriculum policies should address the role of specific subjects as vehicles for teaching students about mental health. Additionally, the role of subjects as vehicles through which students can communicate about mental health is also an important aspect to address when formulating policies.

CASE STUDY

A primary school demonstrated their commitment to a whole school approach to mental health by embedding mental health into the school vision and values statements. In addition, each school policy was revised to include a section on mental health. The assessment policy was amended to take teacher workload into account by reducing marking and feedback. Subject policies included reference to ways of promoting resilience. All staff were given professional development on how to spot the signs of mental health, and information was given to parents on how to support different mental health needs.

PREJUDICE-BASED BULLYING

Schools have a responsibility to uphold the principles of the Equality Act 2010. It is unlawful to directly discriminate against individuals with protected characteristics. These include age, disability, gender reassignment, pregnancy, race, religion, sex and sexual orientation. Bullying is a form of direct discrimination and all schools should have clear policies and practices for addressing all forms of bullying.

LGBT BULLYING IN SECONDARY SCHOOLS

Stonewall's latest *School Report* (Bradlow et al, 2017), a study of over 3,700 lesbian, gay, bi and trans (LGBT) young people aged 11–19 across Britain, provides the most recent evidence on bullying of young people who identify as LGBT+. The key findings from Stonewall are alarming: 45 per cent of LGBT students are bullied for being LGBT at school; 64 per cent of trans pupils are bullied; 86 per cent regularly hear phrases such as *'that's so gay'* or *'you're so gay'* in school and 84 per cent have self-harmed (Bradlow et al, 2017).

While the 2017 statistics suggest that there has been a reduction in homophobic bullying in comparison with Stonewall's 2012 data, more work needs to be done to ensure that all schools can meet their statutory duties outlined in the Equality Act 2010. There is a clear need to provide teachers with further training and education during their Initial Teacher Education programmes, and while they are in-service, to enable them to proactively address the needs of children and young people who identify as LGBT+.

The standard response of referring an LGBT+ young person to counselling can have a pathologising effect by placing the focus of the intervention on the individual, and thus neglecting the contribution that wider structural forces (for example, the curriculum) play in reinforcing marginalised and stigmatised identities. Bullying, harassment and discrimination can result in marginalisation and psychological distress. However, dominant discourses of bullying in the LGBT literature (Payne and Smith, 2013) emphasise suffering and portray LGBT+ young people as 'victims'. Given that multiple identities intersect, this is problematic (Formby, 2015) because one aspect of a person's identity might be wounded, while another aspect might be positively affirmed. It could therefore be argued that the portrayal of LGBT+ young people as *vulnerable* and in *need of protection* might be disempowering (Airton, 2013).

School environments should be critically interrogated to examine the extent to which they promote heteronormativity (or 'compulsory heterosexuality'). This includes both the hidden and the formal curriculum. The absence of LGBT+ issues in the curriculum and the invisibility of LGBT+ identities and experiences in sex and relationships education have been well documented in previous literature (Formby, 2011). Displays around the school, in corridors and in classrooms should demonstrate a visible commitment to diverse relationships and a zero-tolerance approach to homophobia. Stories in school libraries should reflect the plurality of relationships that exist in 21st-century society. All pupils and staff need to be educated about LGBT+ and other identities (such as gender fluidity) and taught to *respect* and *celebrate* all forms of diversity. Addressing homophobic, biphobic and transphobic bullying is essential, but it is not sufficient in itself; it is reactive and becomes a 'sticking plaster'. Instead, educating children and young people (and staff) about respect, discrimination and prejudice demonstrates a proactive response and has greater potential to change attitudes and values.

EMBEDDING MENTAL HEALTH INTO THE CURRICULUM

Some schools are starting to develop a progressive mental health curriculum for different key stages. Through this curriculum children and young people are taught about specific aspects of mental health including topics such as depression, anxiety, self-harm, resilience, bullying and stress. It is important to focus on strategies which may alleviate problems and to be sensitive to students who may be experiencing these issues. It is essential that the curriculum is age-appropriate and that pupils are educated about strategies to manage different situations. The starting point for younger pupils could be the development of a social and emotional curriculum which focuses on feelings and emotions. There is currently no national curriculum framework in England for teaching children about mental health and schools should use this as an opportunity to shape the curriculum to meet the needs of their pupils.

In addition to a bespoke mental health curriculum, schools should consider ways of embedding mental health throughout the curriculum. For example, pupils might be taught subject-specific resilience strategies to help them address challenging subject content. The role of physical activity in promoting physical, social and emotional health is well documented, and physical education therefore plays a critical role in developing positive mental health. Subjects such as science, English and history provide valuable opportunities for learning about race, religion, gender, sexuality and disability, and addressing these topics through the curriculum can help to promote a sense of belonging.

Schools which offer pupils a broad and balanced curriculum are in a stronger position to promote positive mental health. Subjects such as art, music, dance, drama and physical education promote good mental health. These subjects are also an effective way for pupils to communicate about mental health issues using a variety of modes of expression.

Schools have a critical role to play in reducing 'exam stress' that children and young people experience when they prepare for formal examinations. Providing opportunities for revision during school time is one way of addressing this. Teachers also experience pressure for pupils to attain high grades and it is important that they do not transfer this pressure onto pupils.

CASE STUDY

A secondary school developed a commitment to student leadership of school mental health. Students from across the school planned and led a large conference on student mental health. The students researched topics such as depression, anxiety, self-harm, social media use and substance misuse. The students organised the conference and led the sessions and the conference was given high status. Five secondary schools across the Trust were invited to the conference.

IDENTIFYING MENTAL HEALTH NEEDS

Schools play a key role in the identification of mental health needs even though teachers are not trained health professionals. Some schools may use universal screening with all pupils, while others may use targeted screening with specific pupils. Self-reporting well-being questionnaires are a useful tool to support an assessment instrument which is completed by teachers. The validity of survey instruments may be compromised by a range of factors, including events which have immediately preceded the administration of the survey, and therefore it is important to support an assessment of need with observational data, discussions with parents and pupils. Despite this, self-reporting tools are useful in generating a profile of a child's well-being and this can inform approaches to tailored intervention.

STAFF TRAINING

Teachers can be supported to identify the signs of specific mental health conditions, and assessment of needs should always take into consideration the views of the parent(s) and the child (DfE, 2015). When assessing the needs of a child it is important to observe the child in a range of situations to create a more rounded perspective of the child. A range of professional development opportunities are available to schools, including Mental Health First Aid training (see https://mhfaengland.org). A growing number of charities now provide mental health training to schools. These include Minds Ahead (see www.mindsahead.org.uk), Place2Be (see www.place2be.org.uk) and the Anna Freud Centre (see www.annafreud.org).

MONITORING AND EVALUATING PUPILS' MENTAL HEALTH

Monitoring and evaluating pupils' mental health in a systematic way is becoming a priority for many schools. In recent years schools have developed sophisticated approaches for monitoring and tracking pupils' academic achievement over time. Schools are now starting to consider how to monitor and track pupils' mental health in a more systematic way using commercial software packages. The use of a well-being scale is one way of generating quantitative data on specific characteristics of well-being. Software allows demographic data to be entered for each pupil (eg age, gender, ethnicity, in receipt of pupil premium), which then makes it possible to identify trends. This would allow senior leaders to carry out a more systematic analysis by looking for patterns; for example, it would allow them to analyse the relationship between gender and well-being, age and well-being, attendance and well-being, or exclusion rates and well-being. If the well-being scale is repeated at specific points during the year, then senior leaders would be able to identify changes in well-being over time. For pupils who receive specific and tailored interventions, schools will need to systematically analyse the impact of the intervention on mental health outcomes for those pupils.

MONITORING MENTAL HEALTH IN PRIMARY SCHOOLS

Research by the DfE (2017) demonstrated that 65 per cent of primary schools monitor the impact of all mental health provision, 30 per cent monitor the impact of some mental health provision and only 5 per cent of primary schools do not monitor the impact of mental health provision.

EMOTIONAL LITERACY

Students need to support students and staff to express their emotions in appropriate ways. Emotions fluctuate and are dependent upon a range of factors. Students need to recognise their own emotions and the emotions of their peers. They need to know how to support their peers when they are in need of support through listening, talking and referring cases on. All students need an emotional curriculum through which they are educated about different emotions and the effect of their emotions on the people around them.

CASE STUDY

A school needed to develop a way of restoring a sense of calmness after break times. The school decided to introduce mindfulness as part of a whole school approach. As an innovative school that loves technology, the school decided to use *Mindfulness Dojo*, an online application that helps pupils to understand how they manage emotions and develop mindfulness skills. There was a significant positive impact across the school. Behaviour improved in school and pupils also used the video clips to regulate their emotions at home.

DEVELOPING A POSITIVE SENSE OF 'SELF'

+ Positive school cultures contribute to promoting a positive sense of self for all members of the school community.

+ Everyone has a right to feel valued and senior leaders can engender a positive sense of self by recognising the strengths in individuals.

+ Staff who recognise each other's strengths also contribute to a positive sense of self. Adults have a duty to value children's achievements, thus promoting a positive sense of self.

+ Establishing a school culture which promotes a sense of belonging for everyone is also an important way of developing a positive sense of self.

+ Providing frequent opportunities (eg weekly) to reflect on things that they have accomplished that they are most proud of and to identify subsequent priorities that they need to address.

+ Visibly recognising the achievements of students and staff through blogs on the school website, newsletters and displays is a simple way of developing a positive sense of self. Rewarding achievements for pupils and staff is an important way of building a positive sense of self.

BUILDING RESILIENCE

Being resilient is the ability to recover from adverse experiences. Some children (and staff) are more resilient than others. Children and young people need to be resilient in school and at home when they encounter difficult experiences. These include exam pressures, mastering difficult subject content, dealing with negative interactions from peers and dealing with challenging situations at home.

Resilience enables many children and young people to overcome adversity during their lives (Masten, 2001). However, resilient young people do not overcome difficult situations in isolation; they do so with support from the wider social networks to which they are connected (Roffey, 2017). A common understanding of resilience is the ability to 'bounce back' from difficult experiences (Roffey, 2017). While this is an important characteristic, resilience is a multi-dimensional construct (Luthar, 1993); it is possible to be more resilient in certain situations and less resilient in others (Roffey, 2017). In the latter situations, it is important to help pupils to transfer the resilience strategies that they have developed in one situation to another.

CASE STUDIES

RESILIENCE: PRIMARY

One school's journey started in response to the needs of pupils and the community to develop a language for learning and to raise pupils' aspirations

The school developed a curriculum based around Guy Claxton's Building Learning Power – Resilience, Reciprocity, Resourcefulness and Reflection (the 4Rs). Various pupil-led Councils were established in the school to monitor this work. These included the Learning Council, Character Council and the Well-being Council. The pupils suggested the introduction of the fifth 'R' – Responsibility. Pupils identified peers showing the key aspects of the 5Rs in the classroom. These were recorded on a display in the main corridor. The language of resilience was embedded into all lessons and pupils were taught strategies for promoting resilience. In addition, the school measured various aspects of resilience. These included pupils' attitudes towards themselves as learners, 'stickability', their ability to face challenges and the capacity to learn from mistakes.

The impact of the school's approach to developing a resilient curriculum was clearly evident. The school saw significant improvements in pupils' reflections towards questions such as '*I have stickability*', '*I don't give up*' and '*I learn from my mistakes*'. The teachers took the time to focus explicitly on resilience as part of a whole school approach, and staff, pupils and families understood the impact of resilience on learning attitudes. With a focus on pupil voice, this school embedded a whole-school culture which allowed pupils to understand how resilience can help them with challenges in their learning and help them to learn from mistakes.

RESILIENCE: SECONDARY

Adopting a strengths- and solutions-based approach (Roffey, 2017) will help students to recognise what they can do and support them in achieving solutions to things they find difficult. This strategy focuses on helping students to identify goals and to work towards achieving these, while drawing on internal and external resources. A solutions-based approach places greater emphasis on achieving goals rather than overly focusing on the difficulties that an individual is experiencing. Year 10 students were asked to review their feedback on their mock examinations in all subjects and to identify areas where they had been successful. They were asked to review their examination scripts to identify the characteristics of effective answers, specifically paying attention to why marks had been allocated. They were then asked to use the feedback to identify areas for improvement. They were supported to understand that they could use the techniques they had identified in successful answers to improve their responses to questions where they had been less successful.

PROMOTING POSITIVE USE OF SOCIAL MEDIA

Children and young people increasingly live their lives through technology. As digital natives they have grown up within the digital revolution. Consequently, they view technology as an essential tool which they use for a variety of purposes. Social media has now been around for at least a decade and its popularity is shared across young people and adults. Young people use Facebook, Snapchat and Instagram for various purposes, but research suggests that the use of social media is becoming increasingly private (Frith, 2017). For example, they tend to access the technology in private spaces such as bedrooms, and the increasing popularity of instant messaging has resulted in online discussions taking place in private groups. Consequently, parents and teachers may not be aware of the online activities which take place.

TEENAGERS AND SOCIAL MEDIA

According to Frith's research, over one-third of teenagers aged 15 in the UK are 'extreme internet users', ie they spend more than six hours on a typical weekend day on the internet. Additionally, a third of people in the UK were aged six years or younger when they first used the internet (Frith, 2017). In 2015 the overwhelming majority (94.8 per cent) of those aged 15 used social media before and after school (Frith, 2017).

BENEFITS OF SOCIAL MEDIA

Social media use can support development. For example, it can facilitate access to knowledge which can have a positive impact on academic development. Young people may use social media to complete homework tasks or to clarify subject-specific misconceptions. Research suggests that young people value the social benefits of collaborating online and they may use social media for accessing specific forms of information or support (Frith, 2017). They may use social media to develop their identity as a young person. Additionally, social media can reduce social isolation for those who live long distances away from friends. It can also provide a source of support for young people through an increasing number of apps which are now available.

RISKS OF SOCIAL MEDIA

However, despite the benefits there are risks which need to be seriously considered. Lilley et al (2014) reported that online trolling was experienced by 40 per cent of their participants. Spending too much time online can create social isolation by restricting face-to-face interaction. Additionally, young people who spend too long online can experience sleep deprivation and poor sleep quality (Woods and Scott, 2016), which can then impact detrimentally on their concentration and behaviour when they are in school. The PISA research (2015) suggests that the longer people spend online, the more likely they are to experience cyberbullying, and there is evidence to suggest that social media use can impact detrimentally on children and young people's mental health, particularly for girls (Frith, 2017). Similarly, the OECD has found that excessive internet use can have a negative effect on well-being and the Office for National Statistics found that the longer people spend online, the result is a negative effect on mental health. Evidence indicates that the growth in the popularity of 'selfies' and the increasing prevalence of photoshopped images of celebrities and other idealised images of beauty results in body surveillance and lower body esteem (Frith, 2017; Tiggemann and Slater, 2014). Research has also found that girls experience a more negative mood after viewing Facebook compared to exposure to body-neutral websites (Fardouly et al, 2015). Exposure to harmful content online and the risks associated with sharing too much information with others can result in increased vulnerability. An example of this is the increase in websites which promote self-harm, resulting in its normalisation (Daine et al, 2013).

BULLYING AND SOCIAL MEDIA

Bullying through social media is different from traditional face-to-face bullying in that the harmful content is permanently available for others to see and, for the victim, this can result in repeated exposure to the content which can cause psychological distress. Additionally, the harmful content reaches a much larger audience due to the repeated sharing of that content, which can result in further psychological distress for the victim. Research demonstrates that young people are more upset by cyberbullying than exposure to online sexual content and that girls tend to be more upset about exposure to both than boys (Frith, 2017).

Responding to cyberbullying and exposure to harmful content online can be done through individuals blocking perpetrators of abuse or through parents restricting access to digital content. However, blocking access to digital content can restrict the development of digital skills (Frith, 2017) which are so vital in today's digital world. Everyone has a right to access the benefits of being online.

Developing young people's digital resilience is essential so that they are not psychologically damaged through their screen-based lifestyles. Developing a curriculum which promotes digital resilience at all key stages is one way of addressing the issues of social media bullying. All pupils should be taught about the various types of online and offline bullying using electronic devices, and educated about the potential impacts of bullying both on perpetrators and on their victims. The proliferation of cases of high-profile individuals (for example, Members of Parliament and celebrities) who made disparaging comments online when they were younger demonstrates both the permanency of online bullying and the impact of such bullying on their professional lives as adults.

CRITICAL QUESTIONS

+ How might you support all teachers to understand that the mental health of children and young people is their responsibility?
+ What factors can result in a negative school culture?
+ What factors can have a positive impact on the mental health of teachers?
+ What factors can have a detrimental impact on the mental health of teachers?
+ How might schools work in partnership with reluctant parents?
+ How might cultural perspectives affect parents' or teachers' attitudes towards mental health?

SUMMARY

A whole school approach to mental health is important because it will reduce the number of children who require mental health support in the long term. By creating a positive school culture which supports children, young people and staff, fewer will go on to develop mental health difficulties. Developing a systematic approach to universal screening reduces the likelihood that individuals will be missed. All teachers need to understand that the mental health of children and young people is their responsibility. However, the school leadership team will need to give priority to establishing positive mental health for all members of the school community. If the leadership team do not ensure that this has a strong focus, then staff are less likely to accept their responsibilities.

CHECKLIST

This chapter has addressed:

✓ the importance of a whole-school vision, supported by a set of values, which promote good mental health;

✓ the need for schools to eliminate unnecessary teacher workload;

✓ the need for schools to provide a mental health curriculum;

✓ the importance of systematically monitoring mental health provision across a school.

FURTHER READING

Howard, C, Burton, M, Levermore, D and Barrell, R (2017) *Children's Mental Health and Emotional Well-Being in Primary Schools: A Whole School Approach*. London: Sage.

Shute, R H (2016) *Mental Health and Well-being through Schools*. London: Routledge.

✛ CHAPTER 3

TARGETED INTERVENTIONS

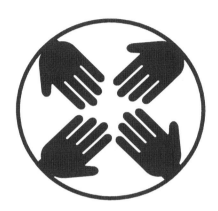

PROFESSIONAL LINKS

This chapter addresses the following:

- The *Special Educational Needs and Disability Code of Practice: 0 to 25 Years* emphasises the importance of early intervention to meet children's needs.

- The Teachers' Standards (Standard 5) places a duty on all teachers to meet the needs of all learners.

CHAPTER OBJECTIVES

By the end of this chapter you will understand:

+ how to identify mental health needs;
+ how different interventions can meet the needs of students with mental health needs.

INTRODUCTION

A whole school approach to mental health focuses on the development of positive mental health for all students. By embedding this universal approach, you will minimise the number of students who need additional interventions. As part of a whole school approach, it will be necessary to develop additional provision for targeted students who require further interventions. You will need a whole school approach to support you with identification of needs. Some students with mental health needs can be effectively supported without the need to access individual or group interventions. Others will require the support of pastoral teams, counsellors, educational psychologists or external services to enable them to thrive. This chapter will address some of the targeted interventions that you can provide in school. Many students with mental health needs do not meet the criteria for referral to Child and Adolescent Mental Health Services (CAMHS) and even when they do meet the criteria waiting lists are lengthy, resulting in support arriving too late. In these cases, additional school-based provision is essential to prevent the problem from escalating.

IDENTIFYING NEEDS

Some students have mental health needs which are both persistent and serious. In some cases, it will be easy to identify these students. They may display visible signs of stress, anxiety or depression, and their social, emotional and behavioural skills may have deteriorated. They may have become withdrawn and a sudden change in mood or behaviour may be evident. These characteristics are not exhaustive but are illustrative of some of the signs that you might easily be able to identify. The signs will vary according to the mental health need itself and to the individual student.

However, it may not be easy to identify all students with mental health needs through your day-to-day interactions with them. Some students become experts in hiding their needs. They may not tell you that they have a need. They may pretend that they are mentally healthy, but the reality may be very different. Some students might choose to 'downplay' their mental health rather than acknowledging the severity of it. The reasons why students might be reluctant to disclose their mental health needs could be due to a combination of factors. These might include:

+ perceived stigma associated with the need;

+ fear that they will be negatively labelled;

+ fear that their parents might find out;

+ fear of negative perceptions by peers and teachers;

+ an internal belief that they are in control of their mental health even when a situation is spiralling out of control;

+ feelings of shame.

For these reasons, it is crucial that schools de-stigmatise mental health by teaching students that:

+ everyone has mental health;

+ mental health falls along a spectrum which ranges from positive mental health to mental illness;

+ mental health can fluctuate and is shaped by our experiences and interactions with others;

+ it is OK to not be OK;

+ there are things that we can do that can make us mentally healthy.

Those students who feel ashamed about their mental health or those who worry about other people's perceptions are more difficult to identify. Internally, they may be struggling to cope but outwardly they may appear to be coping well. Some schools are now screening all students so that all those with mental health needs are identified. Systems to support the identification of needs vary across schools but approaches include:

+ student self-reporting questionnaires;

+ one-to-one well-being conversations with a student once per term;

+ systematic feedback from parents and carers.

PASTORAL PROVISION

High-quality pastoral provision is an effective part of a whole school approach to mental health. It is important that children and young people have someone to talk to if they require support. Some young people do not feel able to talk to their parents or even their peers for a variety of reasons. They may feel more comfortable talking to someone who is neutral. Pastoral workers need to demonstrate the ability to empathise with young people and need to be skilled at listening. Some young people may access pastoral support independently as they may recognise that they need support. Others may have been referred on to pastoral support by a teacher or another adult in school. When young people access pastoral support, we recommend that the following model of listening is applied:

+ Set boundaries: explain to the young person what your role is and explain that you may not be able to keep the conversation confidential. In some cases, you will be able to maintain confidentiality but in cases where young people may be at risk of harm you may need to tell specific individuals who need to be aware of the situation.

+ Ask the child or young person to explain to you in their own words what the problem is. Try to listen to them without interrupting them and maintain a non-judgemental approach. It is important to maintain eye-contact and to consider how your body language and use of non-verbal cues may be interpreted by the young person.

+ Ask the child or young person if they can suggest solutions to the problem. It is far more effective for young people to take ownership of the problem so that they are in control. If they cannot suggest any solutions, then you may need to present the child or young person with several options. However, in this case always seek their opinion in relation to these.

+ Together, develop a strategy or action plan to address the problem.

+ Ask the child or young person to reiterate back to you what has been agreed.

PEER AMBASSADORS

Some young people may not feel confident speaking to an adult. They may prefer to speak to a peer about their mental health. Some schools are training groups of young people to be peer ambassadors. Once trained, these ambassadors can provide a friendly listening ear to peers who need support. If you decide to adopt this approach there are several things that you should consider:

+ Consider which young people might make good peer ambassadors. Peer ambassadors need to demonstrate a required level of maturity. They need to be able to demonstrate patience, discretion and empathy.

+ Develop a programme of training to skill them up for the role. The content of this training should cover common mental health needs, approaches to support effective listening, expectations about confidentiality and when to refer cases on to specific named adults.

+ Consider how much time the peer ambassadors will be expected to devote to this role. If they have examination classes, it is important that the role does not interfere with their own academic development.

+ Consider their caseload so that they are not over-burdened.

+ Consider how you will match individuals to peer ambassadors.

CRITICAL QUESTIONS

+ What are the benefits of being a peer ambassador?

+ What are the disadvantages of being a peer ambassador?

CASE STUDY

A secondary school developed a peer ambassador scheme specifically to support young people through exam stress. Peer ambassadors from Year 11 were recruited to run subject-based interventions and revision classes. These subject ambassadors were the highest-performing students in the year group. They received training in some simple teaching techniques, including modelling and questioning, and they also received training in strategies to reduce stress and anxiety. They ran revision classes and stress-busting classes close to exam time.

COUNSELLING

Not all schools have the benefit of a school counselling service, but many secondary schools now employ counsellors to support children and young people with mental health needs. Counsellors are specifically trained to use counselling techniques, including the use of therapeutic approaches. Young people sometimes self-refer to school counselling services and others may be 'sign-posted' to a counsellor by an adult. Knowing when to refer a young person to counselling is critical. Some mental health needs can be effectively supported without the need for counselling. However, in the case of more severe mental health needs, a young person may require counselling support. The following critical questions should help you to decide whether a referral to counselling is necessary.

CRITICAL QUESTIONS

+ Is the mental health need causing psychological distress?
+ How severe is the need?
+ How long has the child or young person experienced poor mental health?
+ Is the child or young person at risk?
+ Is the child or young person not coping?

Your responses to these questions will determine whether the child needs counselling. Sometimes it is not appropriate to refer a child or young person to counselling. An example of when it may not be appropriate is when a young person declares to a teacher that they identify as lesbian, gay, bisexual or transgender. A referral to counselling in this situation might lead the young person to feel as though something is 'wrong' with them and that they need therapy to make them better. They may resent this and push back against it. In most cases adults refer young people to counselling because they believe that it will help them. Suggesting to a child or young person that they may benefit from counselling should be well considered. In the case of young people who identify as LGBT, counselling may be necessary because they may be experiencing psychological distress due to prejudice-based bullying. If the bullying has resulted in mental health needs, then counselling may be an appropriate option. However, suggesting a referral solely based on a young person 'coming out' may not be appropriate.

● 64 per cent of primary schools do not have access to a school-based counsellor;

● Schools may be left with a funding gap of 10.7 per cent in 2020–22, which will result in schools cutting back on mental health services.

(House of Commons, 2016–17)

CRITICAL QUESTIONS

+ What are the advantages of school counselling?
+ What are the disadvantages of school counselling?

CASE STUDY

A primary school funded a member of support staff to undertake a training course in counselling therapy. The course was part time and required evening attendance for a year. Upon completion of the course, the member of staff was able to provide counselling support across the school. Three other members of support staff were also funded to undertake professional development courses in sand therapy, play therapy and art therapy. This enabled them to deliver interventions within school to specific children.

CRITICAL QUESTIONS

+ What are the advantages of delivering therapies in school?
+ What other therapies might be funded and implemented in schools?

SOLUTION-FOCUSED APPROACHES

Solution-focused coaching is an approach which helps children and young people to develop a positive sense of self. Some children with social, emotional and mental health needs may demonstrate inappropriate behaviour from time to time. In most cases schools use a system of rewards and sanctions, and sanctions are often implemented when poor behaviour is demonstrated. In these situations, the child or young person is usually reprimanded and asked to explain why they demonstrated the undesired behaviour. Additionally, they may be asked to think about the effect of their behaviour on others and asked to identify how they are going to put things right. The problem with this approach is that it reinforces the message within the child or young person that they have done something wrong and this can result in negative thinking.

A solution-focused approach shifts the conversation to a positive discussion. The general principle is that the negative incident is not discussed. The child or young person is helped through skilled questioning to recognise that they have positive character traits. In addition, they are asked to imagine a more positive future for themselves. Examples of solution-focused questions include the following:

+ What do you think you are good at?

+ What do your parents think you are good at?

+ What is the best thing about you?

+ Can you tell me about a time when you did something kind?

+ If you could change yourself to be the best version of you, what would that look like?

+ Imagine making other people extremely happy or proud. What would you do to reach this goal?

+ What makes you a great friend?

+ In sports you have great resilience and team-working skills. You already have these skills so how can you now become a great learner in the classroom?

+ If I scored you on a scale from 1–10 for your behaviour where would you be? Now imagine achieving a score of 10. What do you need to do to move up the scale?

+ You are good at listening to your friends, so you are a good listener. If I scored your overall listening skills from 1–10 what score would you give yourself? What do you need to do to move up the scale?

+ What are your goals for the future?

+ What do you need to do to achieve your goals?

+ What do you want to get better at in the classroom? What do you need to do to achieve this?

One of the key aims of solution-focused approaches is to enable the child to develop a positive sense of self. Many children demonstrate poor behaviour because they have a poor sense of self. In these cases, the situation is unlikely to improve unless you can help the child to improve their self-concept. Teachers, adults, parents and peers are key sources of self-concept and self-esteem. By developing within the child a positive sense of self this will usually have a positive impact on their behaviour. All behaviour is an attempt to communicate, even poor behaviour.

CRITICAL QUESTIONS

+ What are the advantages of solution-focused approaches?
+ What are the disadvantages of this approach?

Systems of rewards and sanctions are based on the theory of behaviourism and B F Skinner's theory of operant conditioning. Skinner believed that rewards should be given for positive behaviour and sanctions should be given for poor behaviour. The general principle of behaviourism is that if rewards are given for good behaviour the child will demonstrate this more frequently, and if sanctions are applied to poor behaviour the child will do this less. The problem with behaviourism is that it addresses the consequences of behaviour and not the causes.

A solution-focused approach is based on the theory of humanism which is accredited to the work of Carl Rogers and Abraham Maslow. This theory emphasises the importance of building a positive sense of self to help the child to achieve their true educational potential. By developing a positive sense of self, children and young people are less likely to demonstrate undesirable behaviours.

PSYCHOLOGICAL SUPPORT

Some children and young people may have severe mental health needs which require the support of a child psychologist. Specific criteria for referral will need to be met including the severity and duration of the mental health needs. Support from child psychologists will usually be accessed through Child and Adolescent Mental Health Services (CAMHS). However, waiting times are lengthy and many young people receive the support too late.

In cases where young people's mental health has had a detrimental impact on their social, emotional, behavioural or academic development, a referral to the educational psychologist might be necessary. Again, it is important to emphasise that specific criteria will need to be demonstrated, for example, the extent to which academic attainment has dropped in comparison with their peers. You should follow the guidance in the special educational needs Code of Practice (DfE, 2015) if you are considering making a referral to an educational psychologist. It is also important to stress that external professionals will usually only work directly with children and young people if parental consent has been sought.

CRITICAL QUESTIONS

+ What are the elements of the Graduated Approach in the *Special Educational Needs and Disability Code of Practice*?

+ In what situations might a referral to a psychologist not be appropriate?

---

50 per cent of mental illness in adult life (excluding dementia) starts before age 15.

75 per cent of mental illness has started by age 18.

(House of Commons, 2016–17)

Research demonstrates that the average waiting time for a first appointment with CAMHS is now six months, and it is nearly ten months until treatment begins. This means that many young people will not receive timely support for their mental health needs and therefore in-school provision is essential.

(British Youth Council, 2017)

SAND THERAPY, ART THERAPY AND LEGO™ THERAPY

Some schools operate a wide range of interventions to support the mental health needs of specific children. These include sand, art and Lego™ therapies. You will need to ensure that specific staff members are trained to deliver these therapies so that they implement them correctly. You will need to source professional development courses that train staff in the principles that underpin each of these therapies. All these therapies are valuable because children are more likely to talk about their mental health or about adverse experiences when they are engaged in meaningful tasks. Young children in particular usually find it difficult to express themselves when they do not have an activity to focus on. Activities such as these will help the child to relax and can provide a vehicle for children to express how they feel using different media. They can also provide a focus for the child as you engage them in discussion about how they feel.

THE VOICE OF THE CHILD

The *Special Educational Needs and Disability Code of Practice* (DfE, 2015) emphasises the importance of consulting children when making decisions about additional and different interventions. The United Nations Convention on the Rights of the Child (Article 12) also emphasises the importance of consulting children in relation to all matters that affect them.

SEEKING THE VIEWS OF PARENTS

The *Special Educational Needs and Disability Code of Practice* (DfE, 2015) emphasises the need to involve parents in all decisions which affect their child. Parents should be asked to contribute to:

+ setting targets for their child;

+ decisions about educational provision;

+ reviews of their child's progress.

SUMMARY

This chapter has outlined a range of targeted interventions which schools might use to provide support to children with the most severe mental health needs. Targeted intervention may be necessary when the mental health needs have started to interfere with the young person's usual day-to-day functioning. Some interventions may be provided by external services and some interventions can be provided in school, providing that staff have been adequately trained to deliver the interventions. In all cases, you should seek the views of the child and parents before implementing additional interventions.

CHECKLIST

This chapter has addressed:

✓ a range of interventions which may be provided for children and young people;

✓ the importance of consulting the child before placing them on interventions;

✓ the importance of seeking the perspectives of parents prior to implementing interventions;

✓ the need to meet strict referral criteria to be able to access external services.

FURTHER READING

House of Commons (2018) *The Government's Green Paper on Mental Health: Failing a Generation.* London: House of Commons.

Shute, R H (2016) *Mental Health and Wellbeing through Schools.* London: Routledge.

✚ CHAPTER 4

WORKING IN PARTNERSHIP WITH PROFESSIONAL SERVICE TEAMS

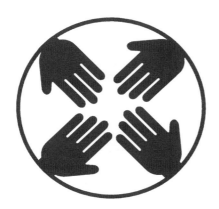

PROFESSIONAL LINKS

This chapter addresses the following:

- The *Special Educational Needs and Disability Code of Practice: 0 to 25 Years* (DfE, 2015) emphasises the need for effective joint working with external services.

- Section 25 of the Children and Families Act 2014 places a duty on local authorities to ensure effective multi-agency collaboration between services for pupils with special educational needs, including those with mental health needs.

CHAPTER OBJECTIVES

By the end of this chapter you will learn about:

+ the roles of professional service teams;

+ the professional challenges that you might experience and ways to overcome these;

+ theories of multi-agency collaboration.

INTRODUCTION

This chapter outlines some of the professional service teams that can support children and young people's mental health needs. It also outlines some of the challenges associated with multi-agency collaboration and information sharing. Schools can do a great deal to support children with mental health needs. However, some needs are so complex and enduring that schools may require support from external professional services to support them in meeting the needs of specific children. The *Special Educational Needs and Disability Code of Practice* (DfE, 2015) has emphasised the need for effective joint working between different services. This is difficult to achieve without a comprehensive understanding of the roles of different professionals who work within wider children and young people's services.

THE ROLE OF CHILD AND ADOLESCENT MENTAL HEALTH SERVICES

Child and Adolescent Mental Health Services (CAMHS) provide specialist support for children with mental health needs. Local CAMHS services are multi-professional teams which include a range of professionals. These include psychiatrists, psychologists, social workers, nurses, support workers, occupational therapists, psychological therapists (child psychotherapists, family psychotherapists, play therapists and creative art therapists), primary mental health link workers and specialist substance misuse workers. Schools can make referrals to CAMHS, but this provision is usually reserved for young people who have severe, complex and enduring difficulties. Schools will need to check referral criteria before contacting CAMHS and any decision to refer children for support must be done with full agreement from the child's parents. Waiting times to access CAMHS services can be lengthy and this can result in young people receiving help far too late. CAMHS does not provide support for children solely with learning difficulties or for behavioural problems which are evident in school but not at home. It is a specialist service for children and young people with severe, complex and enduring mental health needs.

- 5.8 per cent or just over 510,000 children and young people have a conduct disorder.

- 3.3 per cent or about 290,000 children and young people have an anxiety disorder.

- 0.9 per cent or nearly 80,000 children and young people are seriously depressed.

- 1.5 per cent or just over 132,000 children and young people have severe ADHD.

(Future in Mind, 2015)

CRITICAL QUESTIONS

+ Why do you think that waiting lists for CAMHS are lengthy?

+ What actions can schools take to secure a successful referral?

THE ROLE OF EDUCATIONAL PSYCHOLOGY SERVICES

Educational psychologists (EPs) may be employed by the local authority, some work individually and others are employed through private companies. The role of the EP is to provide support for children and young people who experience problems with their successful participation in school. These needs may arise due to learning difficulties or social and emotional problems. The role of an EP is multi-faceted and may include:

+ assessing learning and emotional needs through working directly with the child or young person;

+ developing and supporting therapeutic and behaviour management programmes;

+ delivering professional development for schools;

+ championing the views of parents;

+ writing reports to make formal recommendations on action to be taken, including formal Education and Health Care Plans (EHCPs);

+ attending multi-disciplinary case conferences;

+ developing and applying effective interventions to promote psychological well-being, social, emotional and behavioural development and to raise educational standards.

EPs specifically apply their knowledge of psychology to increase the participation of children and young people in their education. In cases where mental health needs start to impact on learning, behaviour and participation in education, EPs can support schools in developing specific interventions which should improve outcomes for the child.

It is important that schools have comprehensive documentation to evidence what has already been done before making a referral for EP support. This documentation should include:

+ assessments of the child in a range of contexts;

+ details about the evidence-based interventions which have been implemented to address the needs of the child;

+ evidence that the impact of interventions on outcomes for the child has been systematically monitored and evaluated;

+ evidence that the child's progress has been reviewed regularly;

+ views of the child or young person;

+ views of the parent.

Schools will need permission from the child's parents before deciding to refer a child for EP support. The EP will usually write a report and a copy is forwarded to the school and the parents. Schools should consider the recommendations which have been made by the EP and take responsibility for implementing these to secure better outcomes for the child.

THE ROLE OF SCHOOL-BASED COUNSELLING SERVICES

According to the DfE (2016, p 6) *'counselling is an intervention that children or young people can voluntarily enter into if they want to explore, understand and overcome issues in their lives which may be causing them difficulty, distress and/or confusion'*. School-based counsellors help children and young people to gain a better understanding of themselves and gain greater awareness of the personal resources they have at their disposal for managing specific situations. Providing access to a school-based counsellor provides more immediate support for a young person because there is no need to obtain a clinical diagnosis before a child can start to access school-based counselling. Schools may decide to refer a young person to school-based counselling for a variety of reasons, including where emotional and behavioural concerns exist or in cases of bullying. Students who experience academic pressure or other forms of stress may also benefit from counselling.

School-based counsellors tend to adopt a humanistic approach. This means that they tend to demonstrate unconditional positive regard for the young person, regardless of the situation, and they help them to recognise their own strengths. Some school-based counselling services operate through a 'drop-in' service or through an appointments-only system. There are strict professional boundaries between the counsellor and the client, and all counsellors should make these very clear to young people.

School-based counsellors can help young people to work towards goals and increase their resilience. They can support young people to work through relationship difficulties, manage their emotions, and increase their motivation and self-confidence. They can reduce psychological distress in young people and provide support for groups of young people that are 'at risk', including young people who identify as LGBT or those in care.

School-based counsellors can work with the child or young person alongside specialist support provided by CAMHs. They can also provide early intervention to present the need for a referral to specialist services.

Some schools fund school-based counselling from pupil premium funding or from other funding streams in the school budget. School-based counsellors need a safe, private and confidential space in which to work. However, all school-based counsellors need to understand that confidentiality can never be absolute, especially where concerns exist about the safety and welfare of a child or young person.

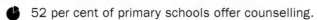
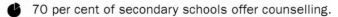

- 62 per cent of schools offer counselling services to their pupils.
- 52 per cent of primary schools offer counselling.
- 70 per cent of secondary schools offer counselling.

(DfE, 2016)

CRITICAL QUESTIONS

+ What are the barriers to establishing and operating school-based counselling services?
+ What are the advantages of receiving counselling?
+ What are the disadvantages of receiving counselling?

CASE STUDY

A school faced increasing mental health needs from students over a sustained period. This negatively influenced attendance, academic progress and the ability of students to engage emotionally and socially with school and home life. Issues included increased incidents of self-harm, anxiety, family breakdowns and problems with friendships.

The school had a good team of professionals including heads of year, the senior leadership team and an effective pastoral support team. However, due to the increasing needs of the young people, the school felt the need to increase the level of support for their students, families and staff to form a more holistic approach to supporting their well-being.

The school set up a dedicated support centre, which was managed on a day-to-day basis by two highly trained and experienced well-being professionals (who were also Designated Deputy Safeguarding Leads). The centre also included the school's Special Educational Needs and Disability team.

The centre worked with children and young people who had experienced problems in relation to participating in learning. The centre worked collaboratively with social services, the police and CAMHS, and provided a bespoke service to each young person to ensure their emotional health and well-being was at a level where they could regain access to their learning and confidently achieve their full potential both in their learning and to become stable, successful young adults. The centre also accessed support from local Youth Support, Educational Psychology, local health and domestic violence services, school-based counselling, Young Carers and Cruse.

Pupils, teachers and parents became aware of the comprehensive mental health provision that the school offered. There was an increase in the number of young people who were prepared to speak openly about their mental health needs and a reduction in the stigma around it. There was a significant reduction in the number of incidents of self-harm and peers were more aware of issues within friendships and were able to highlight concerns about their friends. Feedback from students and parents was highly complimentary about the support that they received, both in prevention of issues and support during crises. Former students continue to access the service on occasion.

Peer mentoring, where children with a problem are paired with those without, has been demonstrated to have a positive impact on the mental health of children with problems (Browne et al, 2004). This facilitates the modelling of different ways of thinking or behaving and therefore this approach might be an alternative to school-based counselling.

THE ROLE OF SOCIAL CARE

Children's social services teams work collaboratively with schools, families and other services to ensure that children can lead safe, healthy and secure lives so that they are able to flourish. Social care services aim to protect children from abuse and neglect. They support vulnerable families in a variety of ways to ensure the best possible outcomes for children and young people.

Schools need to be vigilant. Children and young people who are being abused and neglected may demonstrate signs of poor mental health.

Sudden changes to moods or behaviours should be monitored carefully. If you suspect that a mental health need has been caused by abuse or neglect, then you should discuss your concerns with the designated safeguarding lead in the school and decide whether to refer the case to the Local Safeguarding Children's Board. If the child or young person is in danger, then an immediate referral should be made.

Sometimes, a mental health need may not arise from abuse or neglect, but parents may require additional support in managing this need at home. In these cases, you should discuss with the parent(s) whether a referral to social care might provide an additional layer of support for the family. Some parents may become anxious about a potential referral and fear that the child will be removed from the family. You will need to reassure the parent(s) that this is extremely unlikely and will only occur if the child is in immediate danger. Separating children from their families is a last resort.

THE ROLE OF SCHOOL-BASED HEALTH SERVICES

School-based health services are delivered by qualified school nurses and health care practitioners. School-based health services can provide early intervention and prevent problems from escalating. School-based health professionals can provide an additional layer of support in schools for children and young people with mental health needs. They can provide targeted intervention for a range of needs including support for managing conditions such as anxiety, depression, substance misuse or emotional health. They can provide direct education and targeted intervention on matters related to sexual health. In addition, school-based health professionals play a valuable role in enabling education colleagues to more effectively support children and young people with mental health needs through coaching or other forms of professional development.

CRITICAL QUESTIONS

+ What are the challenges associated with school-based health services?
+ What are the solutions to these challenges?

EFFECTIVE PARTNERSHIP WORKING

Working in partnership with other professionals is complex but it can be rewarding at the same time. Effective collaboration is dependent upon several factors. These include:

+ Child first: placing the child central to the collaboration by always focusing on outcomes for the child helps to ensure that all decisions are made in the child's best interests.

+ Knowledge: having knowledge of the roles and responsibilities of other professionals is essential to effective multi-agency collaboration.

+ Trust: trusting other professionals to fulfil their professional commitments within resource constraints will make it easier to establish mutual respect.

+ Communication: communicating clearly by avoiding discipline-specific language will help to establish a common language which everyone understands.

+ Respect: respecting other people's roles and adopting the guiding principle that all roles are of equal value. This will frame the way you treat other colleagues.

+ Professional boundaries: accepting that there are limits to one's professional role and that support from another professional or service team might be necessary when the limit has been reached.

CRITICAL QUESTIONS

+ What are the challenges associated with multi-agency collaboration?

+ How might these be overcome?

INFORMATION SHARING

Over the past two decades we have witnessed several high-profile cases of children who have died because of the ineffective sharing of information between different agencies. When information is not shared or when information is shared too late there is a danger that children and young people will be placed in situations which are potentially risky.

Data protection legislation should not be a barrier to sharing information in cases where young people are at risk of harm. If you need to share information about a child, where possible you should explain to them why you need to share information, what information will be shared and who the information will be shared with. It is better to get the child's consent but if you believe that a child is at risk you are still able to share the information.

According to HM Government (2015) information which is shared should be:

+ Proportionate: only share the information that is necessary by ensuring that information shared is proportionate to the need to share it and to the potential risks to the child.

+ Relevant: only share relevant information.

+ Adequate: ensure that the information is adequate and enables other professionals to fulfil their professional commitments.

+ Accurate: ensure that the information is accurate and includes facts, not opinions.

+ Timely: information should be shared in a timely way, particularly in cases where the child is at risk or in immediate danger.

+ Secure: follow the school's policy to ensure that information is stored securely.

When sharing information, you will need to ensure that you are compliant with the new data protection regulations (General Data Protection Regulations, GDPR) which affect all organisations, including schools.

CRITICAL QUESTIONS

+ What are the barriers to information sharing between different agencies?

+ How can these barriers be overcome?

SCHOOL BUDGETS

The cuts to school budgets and to budgets for external services in recent years has resulted in services being stretched to their limits, and this has led to schools not being able to afford services such as school-based counselling. One way to address this problem is for schools to fund a pastoral worker or teacher to undertake a short course on a specific approach such as solution-focused coaching. Although a short course would not lead to qualification as a professional counsellor, it would provide them with sufficient knowledge to apply the general principles of the approach and provide professional development to the rest of the staff in these principles. Another approach is for schools to share resources across a multi-academy trust. Schools operating together in a trust can develop local agreements for working with other professional services. Schools also have the freedom to purchase services from private service-providers and this may be cheaper than purchasing services through the local authorities.

THEORIES OF COLLABORATION

Lave and Wenger (1991) developed the idea of 'communities of practice'. A community of practice is characterised by the following:

+ Domain: this is the area of knowledge that brings the group together. All members of the group share an interest in the domain and have expertise in it which they wish to share across the group.

+ Community: a strong sense of community is essential for effective multi-agency collaboration. The community is united by its sense of purpose and commitment to the domain.

+ Practice: while knowledge is essential, communities of practice exist to develop practices and share these across the group.

Research cited in the Green Paper (DfE, 2017) shows that only 68 per cent of schools have a designated member of staff responsible for linking with specialist mental health services. This is likely to have a detrimental impact on multi-agency collaboration. Schools with a dedicated staff member who is responsible for collaborating with multi-professional teams are more effectively able to support children's mental health needs.

CASE STUDY

Students at a secondary school wanted to improve local services for all young people through working with the Clinical Commissioning Group (CCG), the Council Health and Well-Being Board, CAMHS and a local university. The young people met with the Council's 'Voice of the Child Coordinator' to discuss issues around mental health. In addition, they made a film for the local CAMHS service which highlighted their current concerns. The school arranged for the young people to meet with the Chief Executive of the local Mental Health Trust to raise their concerns and perspectives on mental health. Funding was secured for a mental health app and the young people contributed to the signing of the local Youth Mental Health Charter. Attending meetings with the CCG enabled the school to successfully pitch for Mental Health First Aid training for all schools in the area. Through these opportunities young people were offered a chance to meet with people in positions of influence to express their perspectives. In addition, they secured funding to host a student-led Mental Health Conference. A local university worked with the students to produce a mental health app and the university is currently conducting a survey with the young people to collect their views on what they think and what they want in relation to mental health. The school secured an agreement from leaders of the council to prioritise mental health and to meet regularly with the young people.

SUMMARY

This chapter has outlined the contribution that specific professional service teams can make to supporting children and young people's mental health. It has emphasised the roles and responsibilities of the teams and outlined some key principles of effective multi-agency collaboration and information sharing. Where services exist within schools, children and young people can gain immediate support without the need for an official diagnosis. However, we recognise that this is a challenge in some schools, particularly where budgets have been reduced. We have suggested some ways of addressing this problem, particularly in relation to counselling.

CHECKLIST

This chapter has addressed:

✔ the roles and responsibilities of specific external services;

✔ the importance of information sharing;

✔ the challenges associated with multi-agency collaboration;

✔ the facilitators of multi-agency collaboration.

FURTHER READING

Gasper, M (2010) *Multi-agency Working in the Early Years: Challenges and Opportunities*. London: Sage.

Kutcher, S and Wei, Y (2015) *School Mental Health: Global Challenges and Opportunities*. Cambridge: Cambridge University Press.

✚ CHAPTER 5

WORKING IN PARTNERSHIP WITH PARENTS AND CARERS

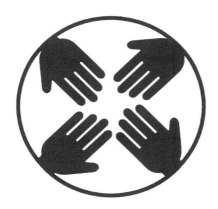

PROFESSIONAL LINKS

This chapter addresses the following:

The *Special Educational Needs and Disability Code of Practice: 0 to 25 Years* (DfE, 2015) emphasises the importance of schools involving parents in all decision-making processes.

CHAPTER OBJECTIVES

After reading this chapter you will understand:

+ how to engage parents in the processes of identifying needs, establishing goals, planning intervention and reviewing their child's progress;

+ how to support the mental health needs of parents.

INTRODUCTION

Throughout this chapter we use the term 'parents' to refer to both parents and carers. Working in partnership with parents is a fundamental aspect of the whole school approach to mental health. This chapter will support you to create effective partnerships with parents. We recognise that developing effective partnerships with parents is not always straightforward. Some parents may be reluctant to engage with the school, while others may be very willing partners. Some parents may have complex needs, including mental health needs, and others may have negative memories of their own education. These factors may affect their capacity to engage with the school. Despite these challenges, children and young people are more likely to thrive when effective partnerships are established. This chapter will help you to address some of these challenges.

SCHOOL CULTURE

All schools should ensure that a non-judgemental, warm and welcoming environment exists for parents/carers. You should aim to create an environment which facilitates a sense of belonging for parents. Outcomes are more likely to be successful if parents and teachers work together to help the child achieve identified goals. Blaming parents for a child's needs is unhelpful and too simplistic. Children's needs often arise from several complex factors which interrelate, and therefore it is unlikely that a need is related to a single factor.

CRITICAL QUESTIONS

+ How are parents treated when they first step into school?

+ Do all staff treat parents respectfully?

+ Do all staff adopt non-judgemental attitudes towards parents?

+ What mechanisms are established to enable parents to express their views?

+ Is there a confidential space for parents to discuss their concerns?

+ Are parents' concerns listened to and acted on?

POLICIES

Parents should have access to school mental health and well-being policies. These should be available on the school website. During the formulation of the school mental health policy, schools should engage in a process of consultation with parents so that parents have an opportunity to influence the policy. This consultation process could be carried out using a paper questionnaire, an electronic survey or using focus groups with parents. The policy should detail the school's overall approach to mental health. Parents should be particularly consulted on the strand of the policy that relates to the school's overall approach to working with parents. They should be provided with opportunities to shape this aspect of the policy. They should also be given opportunities to shape other strands of the mental health policy, including the section of the policy that details how mental health needs will be identified in the school.

CRITICAL QUESTIONS

+ Do you consult with parents when formulating school policies?

+ Do you consult with parents when policies are being reviewed?

+ What are the benefits of enabling parents to shape school policies?

+ What are the challenges?

ESTABLISHING RELATIONSHIPS

Effective relationships with parents should be fostered and maintained. This is particularly challenging in cases where parents express discontent with the school's approach to supporting their child. In some instances, parental concerns will not be justified but sometimes these concerns are well-founded. It is important to keep an open mind and to listen to all concerns. In cases where the concerns are not justified, it is important to give parents time to express how they feel and to calmly explain why their concerns are unfounded. Parental reactions may be emotionally charged and regardless of whether the point they make is valid or not, it is crucial to allow parents to express their views and to take their concerns seriously. In nearly all instances, parents and teachers are striving for the same goals: to enable the child to flourish and to achieve the best possible outcomes. It is important to help the parent to recognise that you are both aiming for the same goals, that you care for their child and that you are doing the very best that you can for them. At the same time, it is important to demonstrate empathy towards the parent, particularly in cases where they have complex needs or face numerous challenges.

COMMUNICATION

All schools should be committed to continuously improving parental communication. Parents should have access to staff or mental health professional/s if they have concerns about their child's mental health. The school should identify a named person who parents can access as a point of contact. In addition, schools should ensure that:

+ parents are consulted during the needs identification process;

+ parents have a confidential space for discussing their concerns with the school;

+ parents who are not able to come into school are provided with other modes through which they can communicate with the school;

+ they respond to communication from parents in a timely manner;

+ communications with parents are recorded and dated;

+ parents are consulted about all aspects of provision which affect their child, including seeking parental permission for external agency involvement;

+ alternative approaches are established for communicating with parents who do not speak English.

INVOLVING PARENTS

Parents should be encouraged to be actively involved in the life of the school. Thus, parents should be fully included in:

+ the initial assessment of needs;

+ planning interventions;

+ reviewing their child's progress;

+ contributing to the school mental health policy.

Parents should be involved in interventions that support their children's mental health and well-being. You should discuss with parents the ways in which they can support their child's needs outside of school. For example, physical and social well-being can influence a child's mental health. Children who are experiencing specific mental health needs, such as depression, may benefit from engaging in physical activity or through participating in social experiences. Some needs can be addressed or alleviated by young people talking through their concerns. Parents play a crucial role in all of these 'interventions' but they might not initially realise that these strategies can have a positive impact on mental health. Your role is to help parents to understand that well-being is multi-faceted and that physical, social, emotional and mental health interrelate. By explaining this, you can help parents to recognise the things they might do with their child outside of school that could have a positive impact on their child's mental health.

It is important that you help parents to understand that mental health is not the same thing as mental illness. Parents need to be supported to recognise that everyone has mental health and that mental health falls along a spectrum which ranges from positive mental health on one side to mental illness at the opposite end of the spectrum. By helping parents to understand that the brain is malleable and subject to influences from the environment, they can start to recognise that mental health can fluctuate in relation to daily experiences which individuals can control.

REDUCING STIGMA

Any stigma shown by parents about mental health should be handled sensitively yet firmly. Some parents may hold negative views about mental health. They may associate mental health with mental illness. Their views on mental health may be culturally influenced or influenced by their own experiences in the past. As teachers we need to challenge stigma by helping parents to understand that mental health is something which everyone has.

It is also important to ensure that staff do not demonstrate stigmatising attitudes towards parents, particularly in cases where parents may have complex needs. Examples include:

+ parents who are alcohol or drug dependent;

+ parents who have mental health needs;

+ parents who have special educational needs;

+ parents who are income-deprived.

As professionals it is not our role to judge parents. Our concerns should focus on the child and how we can work more effectively with parents to enable the child to achieve the best outcomes. While the issues identified above have an impact on the child, we need to recognise that the issues arise out of complex factors which we may not be able to influence. All staff in school should demonstrate empathy towards parents rather than negative judgement. Discussions between professionals and parents should focus on how you can work together to enable the child to flourish, rather than blaming the parents for the child's mental health needs.

CRITICAL QUESTIONS

+ Should schools explain to parents how their needs can impact negatively on their child's mental health?

+ When might it be appropriate to refer cases on to social care?

+ How can schools support parents to support their child's mental health?

+ Do schools have a role to play in supporting the mental health needs of parents?

GUIDANCE AND SUPPORT FOR PARENTS

The school should provide learning, guidance and support for parents to help them:

+ understand children and young people's mental health and its impact on their behaviour and learning;

+ understand the impact of their own behaviour and attitudes on their children;

+ respond mindfully to and manage their children and young people's behaviour positively;

+ understand how to support and stimulate learning at home.

One way of achieving these points is to provide parents with a set of guidance leaflets which provide information about different types of mental health. The information might include signs and symptoms and provide parents with some strategies to support their child at home. Another strategy is to provide a series of parenting workshops on different aspects of mental health and behaviour. Information can be available both in hard-copy and electronic forms and it should also be available in different languages for schools with non-English-speaking parents. Parents should be given information which signposts them to sources of support, including services in the community and online support.

EVALUATING PROVISION

Parents should be provided with opportunities to share their views on how to develop mental health provision in the school. It is good practice to evaluate the mental health provision annually and parental perspectives should be included in this evaluation. A regular cycle of evaluation and improvement planning enables the school to demonstrate a continuous commitment to improvement. Parents should be given an opportunity to share their perspectives in relation to what is working well and what needs to improve. This ensures that parents can contribute to the mental health strand of the school improvement plan.

IDENTIFYING NEEDS IN PARTNERSHIP WITH PARENTS

During the process of identifying needs it is important for schools to capture information about the child's well-being outside of the school. This will help you to ascertain if the mental health need is specific to the school context or whether it is evident outside of school. Any assessment of a child's needs can only be partial if it fails to capture the child's needs in a range of contexts.

You may have concerns about a child. You may have noticed changes in the child's moods or behaviours. You may have recognised that the child is anxious in specific situations. You may have noticed signs that the child is self-harming. It is important to meet with parents face to face to discuss your concerns.

CRITICAL QUESTIONS

The following questions or statements may be useful to help you structure an initial conversation with a parent. In this example we have used anxiety to illustrate how to structure a conversation:

+ *How are you?*

+ *How is George coping at home?*

+ *We have noticed that George becomes anxious in certain situations. These include...*

+ *Have you noticed this at home?*

+ *Why do you think George is anxious? Is there anything that might be causing this?*

+ *This is what we are doing in school to support George... Is there anything else that we could try that might help?*

+ *How do you think you could support George outside of school?*

+ *Let's draw together a plan to support George.*

SETTING GOALS

It is important to help parents to understand that they have a role to play in establishing goals for their child. They should be asked to contribute to goal setting, particularly by identifying goals for their child outside of school. Parents may need support in understanding that goals should be:

+ specific;

+ achievable;

+ realistic;

+ timed.

It is also important to help parents to recognise that goals do not always have to focus on academic aspirations. Goals can relate to social, physical or emotional well-being and parents may need support in understanding how these aspects relate to mental health.

REVIEWING PROGRESS

Systems should be in place to ensure that parents/carers are regularly updated on their child's progress as well as any concerns that may exist. However, effective provision goes beyond merely updating parents on their child's progress. Parents should be actively involved in helping to review their child's progress towards the identified goals. They should be invited to regular review meetings and asked to share their perspectives on their child's progress. In addition, schools could provide parents with more frequent opportunities to share their views on their child's progress. This might involve:

+ creating a paper journal for parents to record their perspectives and to present evidence of the child's achievements outside of school;

+ providing an electronic journal for parents to record their own assessments of their child and to record their perspectives;

+ creating a home-school journal which parents, the child and teachers contribute to.

Electronic journals can be created using free software such as WordPress. This would allow parents to upload a range of evidence, including photographs, videos, blogs and audio files and the child could also add their perspectives. This should not create any additional work for the teacher. Parents could take responsibility for the journal and they could bring it along to review meetings and share the evidence they have accumulated. This is a participatory approach to involving parents in reviewing their child's progress and it would provide them with ownership of the meeting.

EARLY CHILDHOOD EXPERIENCES

Children's early experiences are fundamental to their development and can influence their mental health. Positive interactions with parents in the early years lead to secure attachments which enable the child to feel loved and valued. These interactions enable the child to develop a positive sense of self. Negative experiences can result in the child developing weak attachments with parents, which can have a detrimental impact on the child's sense of self.

52 per cent of children who witness domestic abuse experience behavioural problems and issues with social development and relationships.

(CAADA, 2014)

Early years brain development is critical, and evidence indicates that there is a relationship between brain development and a range of outcomes, including mental and physical health (Spenrath et al, 2011). Early childhood interactions with parents and their experiences in the home influence brain development and adverse experiences can have a negative effect on the child's mental health.

CASE STUDY

All schools experience wide-ranging engagement with parents and unfortunately some parents are reluctant to engage. In some cases, parents may not feel able to share pertinent information, for example, if there has been a history of abuse. Tense relationships can also ensue occasionally between parents and their class teams.

In one school, a dedicated well-being team was established with a capacity to invest time in parental partnerships. The team made home visits during the school day, met regularly with parents, acted as the mediator between the class team and parents (linked but slightly detached), offered advice, shared strategies that worked in school with parents, and became the listening ear for parents.

Impact was evident through improved outcomes for children with mental health needs as a closer working relationship between home and school was developed. Information was shared which might not otherwise have been, and hard-to-reach parents became more engaged.

THE MENTAL HEALTH NEEDS OF PARENTS

Some children and young people who have mental health needs also have parents who have mental health needs. These needs may have prevented them from forming secure attachments with their child. Additionally, in some cases, where parents display mental health needs their children may end up caring for their parent and the parent may lack capacity to adequately care for the child. In some cases, the needs of some parents are so serious that they are unable to provide their child with a safe, caring and loving environment and in these cases, schools may have no choice but to refer the matter to social care. The decision to take children into care should always be a last resort. Schools have a duty of care to ensure that children are protected from abuse and neglect. However, in many cases parents with mental health needs can provide their child with a loving, caring, stable and nurturing environment. It is important that schools adopt a non-judgemental stance towards parents with mental health needs. Teachers and senior leaders should demonstrate empathy and kindness towards all parents, but particularly towards those who are the most vulnerable. Schools can support children whose parents have mental health needs by providing access to an adult mentor. The mentor is a point of contact for a child; it is someone who the child can confide in when situations become difficult at home. Some children may prefer to confide in a peer rather than talking to an adult. Peer mentoring can be effective in these situations. In the case of both adult and peer mentors, it is essential that a positive, trusting relationship has been established between the mentor and the mentee. The arrangement will need to be reviewed on a regular basis to check that it is working. Schools can support parents with mental health needs by signposting them to services in the community which can support them and by providing them with workshops on:

+ stress management;

+ anger management;

+ ways of developing positive interactions with their children;

75

+ strategies for managing depression;

+ strategies for dealing with anxiety.

CRITICAL QUESTIONS

+ What factors might result in parents demonstrating mental health needs?

+ How can schools best support parents with mental health needs?

+ Whose needs should schools prioritise – children's or parents?

Over 2 million children are estimated to be living with a parent who has a common mental health disorder (Manning et al, 2009).

Approximately one in six adults in England will have reported experiencing a mental health problem in the last week (McManus et al, 2016).

From 175 serious case reviews from 2011–14, 53 per cent of these cases featured parental mental health problems (Sidebotham, 2016).

According to Manning et al (2009), parental mental illness is associated with increased rates of mental health problems in children.

Other research indicates that parents of children with an emotional disorder were more than twice as likely as other parents to have emotional disorders (Green et al, 2005).

CASE STUDY

One school had identified several parents who demonstrated signs of stress. The reasons for the stress varied across individuals but included unemployment, debt, lack of stable housing due to financial difficulties, and parents who had caring commitments to other family members. In several cases parental stress was having a detrimental impact on the quality of the relationships with their child. Some parents were irritable, lacked patience and did not manage the behaviour of their child in a positive way. The school decided to host a workshop on stress for parents. This was led by an external provider and all parents were invited to attend. In the workshop, parents were introduced to some practical strategies to help them to manage stress more effectively. They participated well during the session and a follow-on survey indicated that parents were still using these strategies six months after participating in the workshop.

SUMMARY

This chapter has emphasised the role of parents in supporting children with mental health needs. It has also highlighted strategies which schools can use to support parents with mental health needs. Parents should be provided with opportunities to participate in all decision-making processes which affect their child. We have stressed the need for schools to develop a culture of inclusion so that parents experience a sense of belonging and are treated with respect. This will help parents to feel confident and supported. Developing partnerships which are based on mutual respect is not always easy and there may be instances where parents are reluctant to engage with the school or times when parents are overly critical of the school. In these situations, schools should be able to demonstrate that they have reached out to parents by providing opportunities for them to participate. This should not prevent the school from fulfilling its duties towards the child.

CHECKLIST

This chapter has addressed:

✓ the importance of involving parents in identifying mental health needs, setting learning goals, planning intervention and reviewing progress;

✓ the need to involve parents in decisions about school policies;

✓ the role of schools in supporting parents with mental health needs;

✓ the role of schools in supporting children of parents with mental health needs.

FURTHER READING

Berger, H E and Riojas-Cortez, M (2015) *Parents as Partners in Education: Families and Schools Working Together*. Boston, MA: Pearson.

Gorman, J C (2004) *Working with Challenging Parents of Students with Special Needs*. Thousand Oaks, CA: Corwin.

✚ CHAPTER 6

WORKING IN PARTNERSHIP WITH CHILDREN AND YOUNG PEOPLE

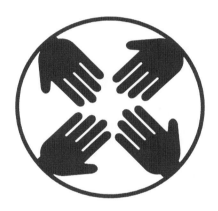

PROFESSIONAL LINKS

This chapter addresses the following:

- Articles 12 and 13 in the United Nations Convention on the Rights of the Child.

- The *Special Educational Needs and Disability Code of Practice: 0 to 25 Years* (DfE, 2015).

CHAPTER OBJECTIVES

By the end of this chapter you will understand:

+ how to facilitate student engagement in a whole school approach to mental health;

+ what student engagement might look like in the context of primary schools;

+ what student engagement might look like in the context of secondary schools.

INTRODUCTION

This chapter considers the role of children and young people as partners in developing a whole school approach to mental health. It addresses ways in which schools can develop these partnerships. This chapter addresses the eight principles of the whole school approach identified by Public Health England (PHE, 2015) but specifically addresses the role of children and young people in the implementation of each aspect of the whole school approach.

THE UN CONVENTION ON THE RIGHTS OF THE CHILD

Article 12 of the United Nations Convention on the Rights of the Child (UNCRC) states that every child has the right to express their views, feelings and wishes in all matters affecting them, and to have their views considered and taken seriously. This right applies at all times.

Article 13 states that every child must be free to express their thoughts and opinions and to access all kinds of information, providing that it is within the law.

The UNCRC is the most widely ratified human rights treaty in the world. The convention came into force in the UK in 1992.

LEADERSHIP AND MANAGEMENT

Mental health provision in schools is more likely to be effective when the mental health of all children, young people and staff is given high priority by the school leadership team. School leadership teams should consider the impact that school policies and associated practices will have on young people's well-being before they are introduced. Leadership teams should consult with young people during the development of specific policies by asking them to consider the impact of school policies on their social, emotional, physical and mental health. One way in which schools can empower students is to develop a student mental health advisory board which is established to advise the school leadership team on matters related to student mental health. The student advisory board can regularly consult other students in the school about issues that affect well-being and they can present these to the school leadership team for consideration.

SCHOOL ETHOS AND ENVIRONMENT

Research demonstrates that the physical, social and emotional environment in the school impacts on young people's physical, emotional and mental health and well-being as well as impacting on academic attainment (Jamal et al, 2013). In addition, research suggests that relationships between staff and students, and between students, are critical in promoting student well-being and in helping to engender a sense of belonging to the school (Cemalcilar, 2010). Key to this strand of the whole school approach is the need for schools to promote a safe environment for all members of the school community. School leaders should promote an environment which facilitates mutual respect.

School leaders should provide opportunities for children and young people to shape the vision, ethos and the physical, social and emotional environment of the school. This will provide them with a sense of ownership and engender a sense of belonging. Providing opportunities for young people to shape the values and rules of the school is an effective way of establishing positive relationships between staff and pupils.

CURRICULUM, TEACHING AND LEARNING

The personal, social and emotional (PSE) curriculum in the school can impact positively on young people's health and well-being as well as providing them with the skills they need (Durlak et al, 2014; Goodman et al, 2015). A comprehensive PSE curriculum should educate young people about how to recognise and manage their feelings, how to cope with conflict and how to support others who might be in need. Schools should provide a curriculum which develops children's mental health literacy skills. This should cover a range of mental health needs including managing anxiety, stress and depression as well as more serious needs such as eating disorders. In addition, all young people should be taught to develop their resilience to adverse situations.

Senior leadership teams can involve young people as co-constructors of a mental health curriculum by asking them to identify the issues that are important to them and involving them in decisions about what they want to learn.

Schools should ensure that all young people are taught about online safety. A digital curriculum should address themes such as cyberbullying and the risks associated with sharing personal information online. The digital curriculum for older children should address themes such as online dating, grooming, sexting, pornography and revenge pornography. All schools should develop a digital curriculum which addresses the development of digital literacy skills, digital resilience and digital citizenship. Children and young people could be provided with opportunities to co-construct this curriculum alongside teachers. Children will be more acutely aware than adults of what the issues are and can be involved in designing lesson sequences to address their concerns.

As well as addressing mental health content discretely, schools should embed mental health throughout the curriculum. Subjects such as art, drama, music and English provide rich opportunities for learning about mental health. Providing children and young people with a broad, rich and relevant curriculum (including extra-curricular activities) which meets their needs is essential for promoting motivation and well-being. Children and young people should be given opportunities to co-create the extra-curricular provision in the school. In addition, a student mental health advisory board can take responsibility for planning how issues of mental health might be embedded through the curriculum. Members of this group could research ways of embedding mental health into specific subjects. Their research could then be shared with subject leaders who could then embed the children's suggestions into curriculum planning.

The physical education curriculum should provide children and young people with opportunities to participate in team sports or individual sports (such as boxing or climbing). These activities will allow young people to develop their resilience as well as having a positive impact on their physical, social and mental health. Young people should be given opportunities to co-create the physical education curriculum with a specific focus on developing curriculum breadth so that all young people are able to enjoy physical activity.

STUDENT VOICE

According to Public Health England (2015, p 14), 'Involving students in decisions that impact on them can benefit their emotional health and wellbeing by helping them to feel part of the school and wider community and to have some control over their lives'. Schools should ensure that children and young people have appropriate channels for expressing their views. They should be consulted about curriculum, learning and teaching, behaviour and assessment policies so that they are able to influence developments which may impact on their well-being. Schools should also provide opportunities for children and young people to form social networks, for example networks for minority groups, and schools should monitor the impact of these networks on their well-being, attendance and academic achievements. Some schools provide opportunities for pupils who identify as LGBTQ to meet informally in a safe, social space. These networks can empower young people and provide opportunities for specific groups of students to influence school policies and practices.

STAFF DEVELOPMENT, HEALTH AND WELL-BEING

All staff in school should be provided with training on how to identify and support pupils with mental health needs. The Designated Senior Lead for mental health should be trained in all aspects of the whole school approach. The nominated school Governor for mental health should be provided with mental health training to develop their knowledge, skills and understanding of a complex area. Schools should seek the perspectives of young people with mental health needs to ascertain what the challenges are and how they can provide more effective support. These perspectives can then underpin staff development programmes. Providing opportunities for young people to input into staff development is one way of empowering them. This might take a variety of forms including:

+ guidance produced by students with mental health needs to support staff development on mental health;

+ students with mental health needs leading professional development sessions for staff;

+ guidance produced by students with mental health needs which is issued to their peers;

+ posters produced by students on mental health.

Some schools are developing innovative peer mentoring schemes where older peers support younger students with mental health needs after they have undertaken a programme of training. These schemes can develop both leadership skills and mental health literacy in peer mentors, and young people with specific needs can be supported by another young person who can offer informal support and advice.

IDENTIFYING NEED AND MONITORING IMPACT

Identification of needs in schools is often unsystematic and relies on children and young people demonstrating symptoms. Once these have been identified, the need is then targeted through intervention programmes to address it. However, many children who have mental health needs do not demonstrate visible symptoms. This means that needs may not be identified and go unaddressed.

There are validated assessment tools which schools can adopt. These include the Stirling Children's Well-being Scale and the Warwick-Edinburgh Mental Well-being Scale. These assessment tools can be given to all children and young people to provide senior leaders with a more accurate perspective on children's well-being. While these tools are primarily self-assessment tools, ie they are completed by young people, they do provide an indication of how young people are feeling at a fixed point in time. This provides leaders with school-level data which can then be interrogated by demographic information such as gender, ethnicity, disability, sexuality and age. Leaders are then able to identify trends (such as differences in well-being between groups of students and whether well-being is declining, increasing or static over time). Standardised resilience scales are also available, and these can be analysed in a similar way to well-being. Standardised tools for measuring attributes such as self-esteem and motivation can also be adopted to enable leaders to obtain a whole-school perspective and to identify children and young people who require specific intervention. The impact of interventions should be systematically monitored using pre-and post-tests. Schools should adopt evidence-based interventions to address the areas of need which have been identified.

The *Special Educational Needs and Disabilities Code of Practice* (DfE, 2015) states that children must be provided with opportunities to participate in decision-making processes. Schools should involve children in the initial assessment of their needs through seeking their views. Children and young people should also be involved in reviewing their own progress regularly and particularly in relation to their perspectives on interventions. Additionally, children and young people should be included in the process of establishing goals or new targets.

WORKING WITH PARENTS/CARERS

Parents, carers and the wider family play an important role in influencing children and young people's emotional health and well-being (NICE, 2013; Stewart-Brown, 2006). A whole school approach to mental health considers the various ways in which a school has the capacity to support parents through information sharing and small-group support. Schools can develop mental health literacy in parents so that they are able to identify mental health needs in their children and provide targeted support where necessary. In addition, schools can also sign-post parents with mental health needs to appropriate services so that they get the help they need more quickly. Schools can also provide workshops to parents on a range of topics including anger management, behaviour management and domestic violence. Effective schools have always worked in partnership with parents to secure the best possible outcomes for children and young people. Involving parents in setting targets for the young person, reviewing progress and providing support at home will foster greater parental participation.

Students should be consulted regarding the school's approach to supporting parents' mental health literacy.

TARGETED SUPPORT

Delays in identifying and meeting emotional and mental health needs can have detrimental effects on all aspects of children and young people's lives, including their chances of reaching their potential and leading happy and healthy lives as adults (Children and Young People's Mental Health Coalition, 2012). Schools should work collaboratively with other professionals to ensure that children and young people get the support they need. The school nurse can play an important role in the identification of needs and they can support the referral process where this is deemed necessary. In cases where pupils receive targeted support, schools should provide regular opportunities for young people to provide their feedback on how effective they perceive this to be.

DEVELOPING PUPIL PARTICIPATION IN PRIMARY SCHOOLS: EXCLUSION

This section addresses this issue of school exclusion and discusses ways of engaging children to prevent them from being excluded. Children in primary schools are likely to be excluded for persistent disruptive behaviour, physical violence and verbal abuse (Gill, 2017).

- 48,000 children are being educated in alternative provision for excluded pupils.
- 55 per cent of 5–10-year-olds in schools for excluded pupils are eligible for free school meals.
- Nearly eight in ten children (77 per cent) in schools for excluded children have recognised special educational needs or disabilities.
- Pupils who leave primary schools with the lowest attainment levels are most likely to be excluded from school.
- Boys are three times more likely than girls to be excluded from school.

(Gill, 2017)

CRITICAL QUESTIONS

+ What factors might lead to a child being excluded from a school?

+ Why do you think more boys are excluded than girls?

+ Why do you think that pupils with low educational attainment at the end of Key Stage 2 are more likely to be excluded than those pupils with higher attainment?

+ Why do you think pupils with special educational needs are more likely to be excluded than those without special educational needs?

Pupils with special needs are unhappier at school, and at greater risk of developing conduct problems, hyperactivity problems and mental ill health (Barnes and Harrison, 2017).

Child mental health has a significant effect on educational progress (Johnston et al, 2014). The more abnormal a child's mental health state, the greater the predicted losses in educational progress (Gill, 2017).

Family poverty has a detrimental impact on educational attainment (Cooper and Stewart, 2013).

CASE STUDY

One primary school identified four children at risk of exclusion. In each case the child demonstrated persistent disruptive behaviour. It was evident that the school system of rewards and sanctions were not working for these children. The pastoral leader decided to adopt a different approach. Following an incident of disruptive behaviour, the pastoral leader worked with the child to identify their strengths. She asked the child to recall a situation in which they had been successful. This was followed by a discussion in which the child was asked to imagine a better future for themselves. The approach was based on the principles of solution-focused coaching. There was no discussion of the disruptive incident and there was no negative tone to the dialogue. Carefully worded questions were used to frame the discussion. These included:

+ How will things be different when the problem has gone away?

+ What things are you good at?

+ How might these things help you to solve the problem?

+ What will you be doing differently when things are better?

+ What will you be doing when things are different?

+ Tell me about the times when you cope better with the problem.

+ Tell me what has worked for you when you have been faced with this problem before.

Over a period of two terms there was a reduction in the number of behavioural incidents for each pupil and the school successfully managed to retain all four pupils.

CRITICAL QUESTION

+ What are the arguments for and against this strategy?

DEVELOPING PUPIL PARTICIPATION IN SECONDARY SCHOOLS: SOCIAL MEDIA

This section draws on the example of social media to illustrate how schools can facilitate student engagement. Some schools choose to ban the use of personal mobile devices due to them being a distraction to students' learning. However, this is a response which negates the significance of technology in young people's lives. We explore here the ways in which secondary schools can work in partnership with young people in relation to mobile technology.

According to the Office for National Statistics [ONS] (2016) the proportion of people using the internet daily rose from 35 per cent in 2006 to 82 per cent in 2016.

The 16–24 age group are the most active social media users with 91 per cent using the internet for social media (ONS, 2016).

More than a third (37.3 per cent) of young people aged 15 in the UK are classified as 'extreme internet users' (Frith, 2017).

Research indicates that young people's online activity is becoming increasingly private (Frith, 2017). It is conducted in their own bedrooms or via a personal smart phone, thus making it more difficult for parents to monitor their children's online activity. Instant messaging via social media platforms has grown in popularity among young people (Frith, 2017) and this has also made it increasingly difficult for parents to monitor online activity. While this may be a cause for concern, consideration should be given to the benefits of social media use for young people.

Research suggests that excessive internet use can have a detrimental impact on life satisfaction (OECD, 2016). The Office for National Statistics has also found an association between longer time spent on social media and mental health problems; 27 per cent of young people who engage with social networking sites for three or more hours per day experience symptoms of mental ill health compared to 12 per cent of children who spend no time on social networking sites (ONS, 2015). Research suggests that young people who are heavy users of social media are more likely to report poor mental health, including psychological distress (cited in RSPH, 2017). Seeing other people online leading idealised lives can result in unhelpful comparisons, which can result in feelings of inadequacy, anxiety, self-consciousness, low self-esteem and the pursuit of perfectionism (RSPH, 2017).

There is an association between sleep and mental health. Poor mental health can lead to poor sleep quality, and poor sleep quality can lead to poor mental health (cited in RSPH, 2017). Several studies have shown that increased social media use is significantly associated with poor sleep quality in young people (Scott et al, 2016). Using social media on phones, laptops and tablets at night before going to sleep is also linked with poor sleep quality (Woods and Scott, 2016; Xanidid and Brignell, 2016).

Research has shown that when young females in their teens and early twenties view Facebook for only a short period of time, body image concerns are higher compared to non-users (Tiggemann and Slater, 2013). The popularity of selfies, the abundance of photoshopped images of celebrities, and the prevalence of 'beautiful' bodies can result in lower body esteem and body surveillance (Frith, 2017).

Cyberbullying is a serious problem which takes a variety of forms. Evidence suggests that it is increasing and that it has a negative impact on young people's confidence and self-esteem (Frith, 2017).

Victims respond in a variety of ways; younger children are more likely to talk to their parents, while older children may talk to their friends. Young people need to develop the digital skills to protect themselves, such as blocking users or updating their privacy settings.

Fear of missing out (FOMO) is linked to higher levels of social media engagement; thus the more an individual uses social media, the more likely they are to experience FOMO. Research suggests that FOMO is associated with lower mood and lower life satisfaction (Pryzbylski et al, 2013).

CASE STUDY

A secondary school had recognised that students were using their mobile devices during lessons to send text messages to their friends. This was highly distracting and negatively impacting on students' learning both for students who were using the technology and those who were trying to concentrate in lessons. The senior leadership team recognised that banning the use of mobile technology would irritate the students. They established an expert student group to research the issues.

The expert group consulted with students and staff across the school. They held a series of focus groups and individual interviews to explore the issues. The expert group decided to use the discussions to also identify recommendations to make to the senior leadership team. The perspectives of students and staff were disseminated back to the senior leadership team by the students.

One of the key recommendations by the students was that students should be allowed to continue to use mobile technology during lessons but only to promote their learning of the lesson content. The next task of the expert group was to draw up a school charter about the use of mobile technology in the school. This identified the roles and responsibilities of the adults and young people in relation to the use of mobile technology. The students felt that this was important because they identified several occasions where staff had used mobile technology for personal use during lessons. The student body was happy that they had contributed to the development of a student charter.

The next task of the expert group was to plan and organise a student-led conference on young people's use of social media. The expert group organised other students to present at the conference and invited a keynote speaker. The expert group led a one-day conference which was targeted at all Year 8 students.

Finally, the expert group developed a social media curriculum for all Year 7 students. This included indicative lesson content, unit plans and resources to support teaching and learning.

CRITICAL QUESTIONS

+ What are your views on banning the use of mobile technology during school time?

+ How can schools work in partnership with young people to address other aspects of mental health, for example stress?

SUMMARY

This chapter has outlined the ways forward for schools to develop a whole school approach to mental health in partnership with children and young people. We have emphasised the importance of consulting young people when school policies are formulated, particularly if policies are likely to have an adverse effect on their well-being. We have emphasised the importance of viewing young people as co-constructors of the curriculum and we have highlighted ways in which young people can contribute to the school ethos and staff development. We have also stressed the role of students as leaders of mental health. Young people are experts in their own lives. Therefore, if we fail to engage them in decisions which affect them we lose their expert insight into the issues which they are experiencing. Forward-thinking schools recognise the contribution that a student voice can make to children and young people's empowerment.

CHECKLIST

This chapter has addressed:

✓ the importance of involving young people in decision-making processes;

✓ the importance of involving young people in establishing goals or targets;

✓ the importance of involving young people in reviewing their own progress;

✓ the importance of developing a whole school approach to mental health in collaboration with children and young people.

FURTHER READING

Department for Education (DfE) (2015) *Special Educational Needs and Disability Code of Practice: 0 to 25 Years*. London: DfE.

Department for Education/Department of Health (DfE/DH) (2017) *Transforming Children and Young People's Mental Health Provision: A Green Paper*. London: DfE/DH.

✛ CHAPTER 7

MANAGING REFERRALS

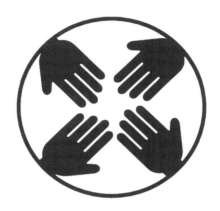

PROFESSIONAL LINKS

This chapter addresses the following:

The Department for Education document *Keeping Children Safe in Education: Statutory Guidance for Schools and Colleges* (DfE, 2016) provides statutory guidance in relation to referrals. This chapter should be read in conjunction with this document.

CHAPTER OBJECTIVES

By the end of this chapter you will understand:

+ when it is appropriate to make a referral;

+ when it is not appropriate to make a referral;

+ the evidence needed to support successful referrals.

INTRODUCTION

This chapter will support you in managing the process of referring children and young people to specialist services. Specifically, it will support you in deciding when it is appropriate to make a referral and when it is not. It will outline the evidence that you may need to present to support a referral and will present case studies to illustrate some of the complexities in relation to referrals. Deciding whether to refer a child to Child and Adolescent Mental Health Services (CAMHS) or social care is not an easy decision to make. In most cases you will need consent from the child before you can even start the process of referral. Parents or others with legal responsibility for the child may also be worried about the implications of the referral process. In all cases it is important to ensure that you place the needs of the child first but you may also need to reassure parents that you believe a referral to specialist services is in the child's best interests. This chapter will provide you with guidance to support you in addressing these issues.

WHEN IS IT APPROPRIATE TO MAKE A REFERRAL?

CAMHS services across England are operating within a period of significant budget cuts and waiting lists are lengthy. Before you take the decision to refer a child to your local CAMHS service it is important to be familiar with the criteria for referral. Although each local CAMHS service publishes its own criteria, there are some general guiding principles which you will need to consider before making a referral. These include:

+ the severity of the need;

+ the complexity of the need;

+ the duration of the need.

In relation to severity of need you will need to consider how serious the problem is. Some problems are life-threatening or place the child at risk of harm and these will need an immediate referral. Generally, CAMHS services will only deal with cases that are severe. Examples include:

+ severe depression;

+ severe anxiety;

+ risk of suicide;

+ risk of self-harm/danger;

+ eating disorders;

+ obsessive compulsive disorders;

+ gender identity needs;

+ severe attachment needs.

This is not an exhaustive list. It merely illustrates a range of needs which may be considered to be severe. Children and young people may present other needs which you consider to be severe. In relation to severity, you will need to consider the impact of the need on the child's mental health and overall life outcomes.

CRITICAL QUESTIONS

+ What are the issues that may arise from each local CAMHS service establishing its own set of referral criteria?

+ The term 'severe' is subjective. One person may consider a need to be severe while another person may not agree. What issues can this create and how might these be resolved?

You will also need to take into account the complexity of the child's need(s). Complex needs arise from multiple risk factors. Specific groups are more at risk than others of developing mental health needs. These include:

+ children and young people who are socially disadvantaged;

+ looked after children;

+ young people who identify as lesbian, gay, bisexual or transgender;

+ those not in education or training;

+ children and young people at risk of, or suffering, abuse, neglect, exploitation or youth violence, witnessing domestic abuse, being a young carer, or having a disability;

+ young people who are in contact with the criminal justice system.

If young people fall into any one of these categories, they can demonstrate complex and often multiple mental health needs. However, young people may fit into more than one of these categories and this can result in several mental health needs which are complex to address and require specialist intervention.

Finally, you will need to take into account the duration of the problem. Some CAMHS services will only accept referral cases where the need has been evident for more than three months. However, judgements about whether or not a specific need is enduring need to be balanced against the potential for harm to the child. It is possible that a mental health need may be so serious that it requires immediate referral to specialist services.

In all cases where teachers or other colleagues have concerns about a child or young person, the designated safeguarding lead in the school should be consulted as they are the person who will usually make the referral. The headteacher and other senior leaders may also need to be consulted. However, when making a referral it is important only to inform those people who need to know. The child's rights to privacy and confidentiality should be respected at all times.

CONSENT

Before making a referral to specialist CAMHS, it is important to discuss your concerns with the parent or legal guardian of the child and to gain their consent for the referral. It is important that parents are willing to co-operate by helping their child to access the specialist intervention, for example by attending meetings. In some cases parents may refuse to give their consent. There may be various and often complex reasons for this. Some parents may be suspicious of therapists and other specialist services, and others may be worried that their child is going to be taken away from the home. It is important to reassure parents that this is an extremely unlikely outcome, unless there are serious safeguarding concerns, and that in most cases it is in the child's best interests that they remain with their family. There may also be complex cultural reasons why some families may resist specialist intervention. It is important to work through these concerns with parents and to reiterate that both the school and family have the child's best interests at heart. Although schools can make referrals without parental consent, it is always better if consent can be obtained prior to a referral as this will increase the chances of intervention being successful.

As well as gaining consent from the parent or legal guardian, it is also important to gain consent from the child. The child will need to under-stand why the referral is necessary and how it might potentially help them in relation to the short- and long-term outcomes. Children over the age of 16 can complete a self-referral if they choose to do so but it is usually more effective for the school, parent(s) and child to agree together the need for a referral. During this process, young people need to be assured of their rights to privacy and confidentiality. While they may agree to a referral, they may be anxious about it and may start to blame themselves. It is important to reassure the child that they are not to blame for the mental health need and that a referral does not mean that there is anything wrong with them; they simply require add-itional support to enable them to thrive. It is critical that schools do everything that they can to remove the stigma that is associated with mental health. Young people may need support to help them under-stand that everyone has mental health, that mental health operates along a spectrum and that mental health can fluctuate depending on one's experiences.

CRITICAL QUESTIONS

+ What factors affect parental ability to give consent for a referral?

+ What factors affect children's ability to give their consent for a referral?

PREPARING FOR A REFERRAL

To maximise the chance of gaining a successful referral you will need to support your referral with:

+ assessments of the need(s);

+ records of interventions which have been implemented to address the need(s);

+ assessments of the impact of these interventions.

You will need to be able to demonstrate evidence of systematic assessment, intervention and monitoring over a duration of time to justify the need for specialist support. Your evidence to support the submission of a referral might typically include:

+ observations of the child or young person in a range of contexts;

+ the triggers which may result in a mental health need;

+ the child's or young person's family context;

+ the impact of the mental health need(s) on attendance, exclusion and academic attainment;

+ specific assessments on the mental health need using robust assessment tools;

+ the views of the child or young person;

+ the views of the legal guardian(s).

You will need to demonstrate that a programme of interventions has been implemented to address the area of need. You will also need to demonstrate that the impact of interventions has been monitored and that interventions have been evaluated and modified as a result of on-going assessments. In cases where interventions are less effective, you will need to demonstrate that different interventions have been implemented and evaluated. Keeping detailed records will maximise your chances of obtaining a successful referral.

There are approximately 460,000 referrals per year to children and young people's mental health services.

200,000 of these go on to receive treatment.

In 2016/17 the average wait for treatment in a children and young people's mental health service was 12 weeks.

(DfE/DH, 2017)

According to research, mental health programmes delivered in school that involve a qualified mental health professional are more effective than those led by teachers (Calear and Christensen, 2010). This supports the case for multi-professional involvement in the delivery of interventions in schools.

CASE STUDY

Lewis was assigned a male identity at birth but from the age of eight he knew that he wanted to be female. Initially, Lewis did not tell his parents, peers or teachers but before he started secondary school he decided that he wanted to be known as Lucy upon transition from Year 6 to Year 7. Immediately prior to starting secondary school, in the summer vacation, Lucy told her parents that she identified as trans-gender. Her parents were shocked and extremely resistant, and refused to use her preferred name. They contacted the secondary school and asked the school to use the name Lewis. On the first day at secondary school, Lucy had a meeting with the Head of Year 7 and communicated her wish to be known by her preferred name. She had also informed all of her friends about her transgender identity over the summer vacation. The Head of Year was very supportive and communicated Lucy's pre-ferred name to all teachers. Lucy's friends were also very supportive. However, her parents were resistant and insisted that Lucy wore male clothing. Lucy had to leave the house wearing male clothing and change when she arrived at school. She had to get changed again before she left for home.

By January, Lucy had become extremely depressed. She had started to self-harm and she craved the support of her parents. Her confidence was declining and her academic grades did not reflect her capabilities. The school had provided Lucy with counselling support, at her request, even though her parents had not given their permission for this to take place. In one counselling session Lucy told the counsellor that she was suicidal. She attributed this to the sense of rejection she had felt as a result of her parents' attitude towards her transgender status. She reported that she could not concentrate in class, that she cried herself to sleep every night and that she did not want to wake up each morning.

CRITICAL QUESTIONS

+ Do you think, in Lucy's case, that a referral to specialist CAMHS is appropriate?

+ What more might the school do to support Lucy?

+ What are your views in relation to the reactions of Lucy's parents?

WHEN IS IT NOT APPROPRIATE TO MAKE A REFERRAL?

Referrals to CAMHS are not appropriate in cases where children and young people demonstrate a typical reaction to a significant life event. These events may include:

+ parental separation;

+ bereavement of a friend or relative;

+ transition to a new school;

+ transition to a new teacher;

+ transition to a new home.

This is not an exhaustive list. It merely serves to illustrate that some needs are usual responses to traumatic or difficult situations. The child's needs can often be supported in school through pastoral support, educational psychology support or school-based counselling. The trigger for a referral will usually be when the mental health need is severe, complex and enduring. However, while some needs can subside or be met through school-based provision, it is important to remember that children will respond to similar experiences in very different ways. For example, while for some children parental separation may result in low mood, for others it may result in self-harm, severe depression or risk of suicide. Decisions about whether or not a referral is appropriate should be based not on the child's experiences, but on the impact that these experiences have had on their mental health.

CAMHS will not usually take on cases where children and young people demonstrate difficulties which only occur in school, for example where a child demonstrates conduct disorder in school but where this is not evident in the home. Therefore, it is important to capture the perspectives of parents who will be able to give you additional information on the child's needs within the context of the family.

CRITICAL QUESTIONS

+ What is the likely impact of parental separation on children and young people's mental health and educational outcomes?

+ What other examples can you think of that might not constitute a referral?

● 61 per cent of schools offer school-based counselling (84 per cent of secondary schools, 56 per cent of primaries).

● 68 per cent of schools have a designated member of staff responsible for linking with specialist mental health services.

(DfE/DH, 2017)

Research demonstrates that socio-economic status affects health, cognitive, educational and socio-emotional outcomes in children (Bradley and Corwyn, 2002). Socio-economic deprivation is recognised across the world as one of the key risk factors which impacts detrimentally on mental health (Patel et al, 2008).

CRITICAL QUESTIONS

+ What are the advantages and disadvantages of delivering mental health interventions in schools?

+ What are the advantages and disadvantages of delivering mental health interventions to children and young people in clinics?

CASE STUDY

Saima is in Year 4. Her parents had recently separated after nine months of domestic violence. Saima's mother was the victim and her father was the perpetrator. During this period of time Saima had witnessed physical and verbal abuse. She was frightened of her father and had experienced significant sleep deprivation. One night, following a domestic violence episode, Saima and her mother fled to a refuge. Saima was terrified that her father would find them and that he would turn up at the school to take her. Saima's teachers had recognised that Saima was experiencing crippling anxiety. She was frightened to go out in the playground in case her father was outside the school perimeter and she worried every day that he would be waiting for her outside of school. The anxiety was beginning to affect Saima's academic perform-ance. Her concentration in class was low and she lacked motivation. She also appeared to be extremely depressed. The school responded by providing pastoral support for Saima. Saima received support during these sessions to help her to manage her anxiety.

CRITICAL QUESTIONS

+ Do you think the school should make a referral to CAMHS?
+ What other support might the school put into place to support Saima?

WHAT EVIDENCE DO YOU NEED TO SUPPORT A REFERRAL?

To support the case for a referral you will need to demonstrate the severity of the need, including the impact of the need on the child's well-being. You will need to include within your referral submission evidence of the impact of the mental health need on the child. This could include the impact of the need on the child's:

+ educational achievement;
+ well-being;
+ behaviour, including risk-taking;

+ attendance;

+ punctuality;

+ sense of self;

+ confidence;

+ motivation;

+ participation/engagement.

You will need to demonstrate that the problem is severe and enduring. Depending on the need, you could submit a range of forms of evidence, including quantitative and qualitative data. Examples might include observations of the child or young person, recent assessments in curriculum areas, absence and exclusion rates, the perspectives of the child and the perspectives of the parent or legal guardian. In most cases, there will be an expectation that school-based support has been implemented, monitored and evaluated. In cases where there has been involvement from other professionals (for example, pastoral staff, counsellors, educational psychologists, behaviour support workers) it will be important to include reports from these professionals to support the case. You will need to demonstrate that you have worked collaboratively with the child and parents during the school-based support phase, and in cases where parents have not engaged it will be necessary to document what steps have been taken to facilitate parental participation.

In cases of children and young people at risk of, or suffering, abuse, neglect, exploitation or youth violence, witnessing domestic abuse, or being a young carer, you will need to make a decision about whether to refer a case to social care. However, these children are also at risk of developing mental health needs, so it might be necessary to refer a single case to both social care and mental health services. All services involved with a child or young person will need to collaborate by sharing information and developing clear lines of communication.

CRITICAL QUESTIONS

+ What are the barriers to effective multi-agency collaboration?

+ What are the facilitators of effective multi-agency collaboration?

SUMMARY

This chapter has outlined the range of evidence that schools might be required to submit to support a case referral to specialist mental health services. It has emphasised when it might be appropriate to refer a child or young person to CAMHS and when it might not be appropriate to do so. It has highlighted the complex nature of some mental health needs and discussed the need to refer some cases to more than one service.

CHECKLIST

This chapter has addressed:

- ✓ the need to evidence the severity of a mental health need when making a referral;
- ✓ the need to emphasise the duration of a mental health need when making a referral;
- ✓ the need to emphasise the complex nature of needs when making referrals, particularly by highlighting the role of multiple risk factors;
- ✓ the importance of gaining consent from children, young people and parents prior to making a referral;
- ✓ the need to include the perspectives of children, young people and parents in a submission for a referral;
- ✓ the need to include evidence from professionals who have been involved in school-based intervention.

FURTHER READING

Department for Education (DfE) (2015) *Special Educational Needs and Disability Code of Practice: 0 to 25 Years*. London: DfE.

Department for Education/Department of Health (DfE/DH) (2017) *Transforming Children and Young People's Mental Health Provision: A Green Paper*. London: DfE/DH.

✛ CONCLUSION

WAYS FORWARD

This book has considered the role of schools in supporting children and young people's mental health. While it must be acknowledged that education professionals are not experts in health matters, schools can play an important role in promoting positive mental health. A whole school approach to mental health should reduce the numbers of young people requiring specialist provision from the health sector. Schools already play a critical role in identifying needs and providing young people with appropriate support. There are examples of best practice across the sector which need to be disseminated more widely. However, supporting children and young people in need is only part of the solution. Effective whole school approaches to mental health promote positive well-being and develop mental health literacy across all members of the school community. This book addresses the eight principles of the whole school approach identified by Public Health England (PHE, 2015).

Mental health provision in schools is more likely to be effective when the mental health of all children, young people and staff is given high priority by the school leadership team. The recent Green Paper, *Transforming Children and Young People's Mental Health Provision* (DH/ DfE, 2017) highlights the importance of the leadership and management of mental health provision in schools through the recommendation that all schools should have Designated Senior Leaders for Mental Health. This is a specialist role which should have parity to the role of the Special Educational Needs Co-ordinator (SENCO). We believe that the role should be given to individuals who have undertaken specialist training in mental health which is accredited at Level 7 of the National Qualifications Framework. In addition, the Department of Health and Department for Education should consult the sector to develop a set of standards to be associated with the role. Like health professionals, such as counsellors, who benefit from mandatory professional supervision, the school mental health lead should be provided with regular supervision from an appropriately qualified supervisor who is external to the school. These recommendations help to signify the importance of the role and ensure that a minimum standard of service is provided across the school sector.

The Designated Senior Leader for Mental Health would be responsible for developing universal provision for mental health, not just for children and young people in need, but for the whole school community. They would be responsible for developing policies and improvement plans to support the implementation of all elements of the whole school approach outlined in this book. Additionally, all schools should demonstrate their strategic commitment to mental health by appointing a named Governor who would hold responsibility for monitoring the quality of the mental health provision across the school. The Mental Health Governor would be responsible for holding Designated Senior Leaders of Mental Health to account.

Research demonstrates that the physical, social and emotional environment in the school impacts on young people's physical, emotional and mental health and well-being as well as impacting on academic attainment (Jamal et al, 2013). In addition, research suggests that relationships between staff and students, and between students, are critical in promoting student well-being and in helping to engender a sense of belonging to the school (Cemalcilar, 2010). Key to this strand of the whole school approach is the need for schools to promote a safe environment for all members of the school community. School leaders should promote an environment which facilitates mutual respect. Policies and practices should be developed for supporting behaviour for . learning, and all forms of bullying should be challenged and addressed in accordance with school policies. In addition to ensuring the safety of all members of the school community, schools should develop proactive responses by educating children and young people about bullying, discrimination and diversity to prepare young people for their responsibilities as citizens to the diverse communities in which they live. Schools should develop policies and practices which promote student voice and all adults should adopt the principle of unconditional positive regard to all children and young people.

The personal, social and emotional (PSE) curriculum in the school can impact positively on young people's health and well-being as well as providing them with the skills they need (Durlak et al, 2014; Goodman et al, 2015). A comprehensive PSE curriculum should educate young people about how to recognise and manage their feelings, how to cope with conflict and how to support others who might be in need. Schools should provide a curriculum which develops children's mental health literacy skills. This should cover a range of mental health needs including managing anxiety, stress and depression as well as more serious needs such as eating disorders. In addition, all young people should be taught to develop their resilience to adverse situations.

We believe that as well as addressing mental health content discretely, schools should embed mental health throughout the curriculum. Subjects such as art, drama, music and English provide rich opportunities for learning about mental health. Providing children and young people with a broad, rich and relevant curriculum (including extra-curricular activities) which meets their needs is essential for promoting motivation and well-being. The physical education curriculum should provide children and young people with opportunities to participate in team sports or individual sports. These activities will allow young people to develop their resilience as well as having a positive impact on their physical, social and mental health.

According to Public Health England (2015, p 14), *'Involving students in decisions that impact on them can benefit their emotional health and wellbeing by helping them to feel part of the school and wider community and to have some control over their lives'*. Schools should ensure that children and young people have appropriate channels for expressing their views. They should be consulted about curriculum, learning and teaching, and behaviour and assessment policies so that they are able to influence developments which may impact on their well-being. Schools should also provide opportunities for children and young people to form social networks, for example networks for minority groups, and monitor the impact of these networks on their well-being, attendance and academic achievements.

All staff in school should be provided with training on how to identify and support pupils with mental health needs. The Designated Senior Lead for mental health should be trained in all aspects of the whole school approach. The nominated school Governor for mental health should be provided with mental health training to develop their knowledge, skills and understanding of a complex area. We are aware that some schools are developing innovative peer mentoring schemes where older peers support younger students with mental health needs after they have undertaken a programme of training. These schemes can develop both leadership skills and mental health literacy in peer mentors, and young people with specific needs can be supported by another young person who can offer informal support and advice.

Identification of needs in schools is often unsystematic and relies on children and young people demonstrating symptoms. Once these have been identified, the need is then targeted through intervention programmes to address the need. However, many children who have mental health needs do not demonstrate visible symptoms. This means that needs may not be identified and go unaddressed.

There are validated assessment tools which schools can adopt to support identification of needs. These include the Stirling Children's Well-being Scale and the Warwick-Edinburgh Mental Well-being Scale. These assessment tools can be given to all children and young people to pro-vide senior leaders with a more accurate perspective on children's well-being. While these tools are primarily self-assessment tools, ie they are completed by young people, they do provide an indication of how young people are feeling at a fixed point in time. This provides leaders with school-level data which can then be interrogated by demographic infor-mation such as gender, ethnicity, disability, sexuality and age. Leaders are then able to identify trends (such as differences in well-being between groups of students and whether well-being is declining, increasing or static over time). Standardised resilience scales are also available, and these can be analysed in a similar way to well-being. Standardised tools for measuring attributes such as self-esteem and motivation can also be adopted to enable leaders to gather a whole-school perspective and to identify children and young people who require specific intervention. The impact of interventions should be systematically monitored using pre-and post-tests. Schools should adopt evidence-based interventions to address the areas of need which have been identified.

Parents, carers and the wider family play an important role in influ-encing children and young people's emotional health and well-being (NICE, 2013; Stewart-Brown, 2006). A whole school approach to mental health considers the various ways in which a school has the capacity to support parents through information sharing and small-group support. Schools can develop mental health literacy in parents so that they are able to identify mental health needs in their children and provide targeted support where necessary. In addition, schools can also sign-post parents with mental health needs to appropriate services so that they get the help they need more quickly. Schools can also provide workshops to parents on a range of themes including anger manage-ment, behaviour management and domestic violence. Effective schools have always worked in partnership with parents to secure the best possible outcomes for children and young people. Involving parents in setting targets for the young person, reviewing progress and providing support at home will foster greater parental participation.

Delays in identifying and meeting emotional and mental health needs can have detrimental effects on all aspects of children and young people's lives, including their chances of reaching their potential and leading happy and healthy lives as adults (Children and Young People's

Mental Health Coalition, 2012). Schools should work collaboratively with other professionals to ensure that children and young people get the support they need. The school nurse can play an important role in the identification of needs and they can support the referral process where this is deemed necessary.

The proposal to introduce Mental Health Support Teams in the Mental Health Green Paper (DH/DfE, 2017) is a positive step because it will enable more young people to get the specialist support they need in school (such as counselling or therapy) and it will minimise the number of children who will require specialist support from the Child and Adolescent Support Services. However, it is critical that these roles are filled by professionals who have experience of working with children in school settings and it is essential that these professionals have undertaken a specialist programme of training relating to specific interventions.

This book has outlined the way forward for schools in relation to supporting children and young people's mental health. Schools now need to become skilled in tracking and monitoring children's mental health with the same rigour that they currently track and monitor academic attainment. Providing specialist input for young people with identified needs is necessary but not sufficient. Adopting a whole school approach will ensure that schools can foster positive mental health for every child and young person.

✚ REFERENCES

Airton, L (2013)
Leave Those Kids Alone: On the Conflation of School Homophobia and Suffering Queers. *Curriculum Inquiry*, 43(5): 532–62.

Aldridge, J M and McChesney, K (2018)
The Relationships Between School Climate and Adolescent Mental Health and Wellbeing: A Systematic Literature Review. *International Journal Of Educational Research*, 88: 121–45.

Barber, S, (2012)
Time to Stop Stigmatising Mental Health Problems at School. [online] Available at: www.theguardian.com/teacher-network/teacher-blog/2012/apr/14/mental-health-stigma-school (accessed 8 August 2018).

Barnes, M and Harrison, R (2017)
The Wellbeing of Secondary School Pupils with Special Educational Needs. London: DfE.

Blum, R W and Libbey, H P (2004)
School Connectedness: Strengthening Health and Education Outcomes for Teenagers. *Journal of School Health*, 74(7): 231–3.

Bor, W, Dean, A J, Najman, J and Hayatbakhsh, R (2014)
Are Child and Adolescent Mental Health Problems Increasing in the 21st Century? A Systematic Review. *Australian and New Zealand Journal of Psychiatry*, 48: 606–16.

Bradley, R H and Corwyn, R F (2002)
Socioeconomic Status and Child Development. *Annual Review of Psychology*, 53: 371–99.

Bradlow, J, Bartram, F and Guasp, A (2017)
School Report: The Experiences of Lesbian, Gay, Bi and Trans Young People in Britain's Schools in 2017. [online] Available at: www.stonewall.org.uk/sites/default/files/the_school_report_2017.pdf (accessed 8 August 2018).

British Youth Council (2017)
A Body Confident Future. London: British Youth Council.

Browne, G, Gafni, A, Roberts, J, Byrne, C and Majumdar, G (2004)

Effective/Efficient Mental Health Programs for School-age Children: A Synthesis of Reviews. *Social Science and Medicine*, 58(7): 1367–84.

Burton, M (2014)

Children and Young People's Mental Health, in Burton, M, Pavord, E and Williams, B (eds) *An Introduction to Child and Adolescent Mental Health* (pp 1–38). London: Sage.

Butcher, J (2010)

Children and Young People as Partners in Health and Well-being, in Aggleton, P, Dennison, C and Warwick, I (eds) *Promoting Health and Well-Being Through Schools* (pp 119–33). Abingdon: Routledge.

CAADA (2014)

In Plain Sight: The Evidence From Children Exposed to Domestic Abuse. [online] Available at: www.safelives.org.uk/sites/default/files/resources/In_plain_sight_the_evidence_from_children_exposed_to_domestic_abuse.pdf (accessed 8 August 2018).

Calear, A L and Christensen, H (2010)

Systematic Review of School-based Prevention and Early Intervention Programs for Depression. *Journal of Adolescence*, 33(3): 429–38.

Cemalcilar, Z (2010)

Schools as Socialisation Contexts: Understanding the Impact of School Climate Factors on Students' Sense of School Belonging. *Applied Psychology*, 59(2): 243–72.

Children and Young People's Mental Health Coalition (2012)

Resilience and Results: How to Improve the Emotional and Mental Wellbeing of Children and Young People in Your School. London: Children and Young People's Mental Health Coalition.

Clausson, E and Berg, A (2008)

Family Intervention Sessions: One Useful Way to Improve School Children's Mental Health. *Journal of Family Nursing*, 14: 289–312.

Cooper, K and Stewart, K (2013)

Does Money Affect Children's Outcomes? A Systematic Review. [online] Available at: www.jrf.org.uk/report/does-money-affect-children%E2%80%99s-outcomes (accessed 8 August 2018).

Cushman, P, Clelland, T and Hornby, G (2011)

Health-Promoting Schools and Mental Health Issues: A Survey of New Zealand Schools. *Pastoral Care in Education*, 29: 247–60.

Daine, K, Hawton, K, Singaravelu, V, Stewart, A, Simkin, S and Montgomery P (2013)

The Power of the Web: A Systematic Review of Studies of the Influence of the Internet on Self-Harm and Suicide in Young People. PLoS ONE, 8(10): e77555. https://doi.org/10.1371/journal.pone.0077555

Danby, G and Hamilton, P (2016)

Addressing the 'Elephant in the Room. The Role of the Primary School Practitioner in Supporting Children's Mental Well-Being. *Pastoral Care in Education*, 34(2): 90–103.

Department for Education (DfE) (2015)

Special Educational Needs and Disability Code of Practice: 0 to 25 Years. London: DfE.

Department for Education (DfE) (2016)

Mental Health and Behaviour in Schools: Departmental Advice for School Staff. London: DfE.

Department for Education/Department of Health (DfE/DH) (2017)

Transforming Children and Young People's Mental Health Provision: A Green Paper. London: DfE/DH.

Department of Health (DH) (2014)

Future in Mind: Promoting, Protecting and Improving our Children and Young People's Mental Health and Wellbeing. London: DH.

Dickins, M (2014)

A to Z of Inclusion in Early Childhood. Berkshire: Open University Press.

Dodge, R, Daly, A P, Huyton, J and Sanders, L D (2012)

The Challenge of Defining Wellbeing. *International Journal of Wellbeing*, 2(3): 222–35.

Durlak, J A, Weissberg, R, Dymnicki, A, Taylor, R and Schellinger K (2011)

The Impact of Enhancing Students' Social and Emotional Learning: A Meta-analysis of School-based Universal Interventions. *Child Development*, 82(1): 405–32.

Ecclestone, K (2014)

Stop This Educational Madness: It's Time to Resist Calls for More Mental-Health Interventions in Education. [online] Available at: www.spiked-online.com/newsite/article/stothiseducational-madness/15382#.VmtXUGcrGM8 (accessed 8 August 2019).

Ecclestone, K (2015)

Well-Being Programmes in Schools Might be Doing Children More Harm than Good. [online] Available at: http://theconversation.com/well-being-programmes-in-schools-might-be-doing-children-more-harm-than-good-36573 (accessed 8 August 2018).

Education Support Partnership (2017)

Health Survey 2017 The Mental Health and Wellbeing of Education Professionals in the UK. London: Education Support Partnership.

Fardouly, J, Diedrichs, P C, Vartanian, L and Halliwell, E (2015)

Social Comparisons on Social Media: The Impact of Facebook on Young Women's Body Image Concerns and Mood. *Body Image*, 13: 38–45.

Formby, E (2011)

Sex and Relationships Education, Sexual Health, and Lesbian, Gay and Bisexual Sexual Cultures: Views from Young People. *Sex Education*, 11(3): 255–66.

Formby, E (2015)

Limitations of Focussing on Homophobic, Biphobic and Transphobic 'Bullying' to Understand and Address LGBT Young People's Experiences Within and Beyond School. *Sex Education*, 15(6): 626–40.

Frith, E (2017)

Social Media and Children's Mental Health: A Review of the Evidence. London: Education Policy Institute.

Future in Mind (2015)

Future in Mind: Promoting, Protecting and Improving our Children and Young People's Mental Health and Wellbeing. London: Department for Health and NHS England.

Gill, K (2017)

Making the Difference: Breaking the Link Between School Exclusion and Social Exclusion. London: IPPR.

Glazzard, J (2018)

Teacher Mental Health. [online] Available at: https://jglazzardblog.wordpress.com/2018/01/07/teacher-mental-health (accessed 3 August 2018).

Glover, S, Burns, J, Butler, H and Patton, G (1998)

School Environments and the Emotional Wellbeing of Young People. *Family Matters*, 49: 11–16.

Goodman, A, Joshi, H, Nasim B and Tyler C (2015)

Social and Emotional Skills in Childhood and Their Long-term Effects on Adult Life. London: UCL.

Green, H, McGinnity, A, Meltzer, H, Ford, T and Goodman, R (2005)
Mental Health of Children and Young People in Great Britain, 2004. London: ONS.

Greenberg, M T, Weissberg, R P, O'Brien, M U, Zins, J E, Fredericks, L and Resnick, H (2003)
Enhancing School-Based Prevention and Youth Development Though Coordinated Social, Emotional, and Academic Learning. *American Psychologist,* 58: 466–74.

Gumora, G and Arsenio, W F (2002)
Emotionality, Emotion Regulation, and School Performance in Middle School Children. *Journal of School Psychology,* 40: 395–413.

HM Government (2015)
Information Sharing: advice for practitioners providing safeguarding services to children, young people, parents and carers. [online] Available at: https://assets.publishing.service.gov.uk/government/uploads/system/uploads/attachment_data/file/721581/Information_sharing_advice_practitioners_safeguarding_services.pdf (accessed 8 August 2018).

Holmstrom, R (2013)
Families, Disability and Mental Health, in Knowles, G and Holmstrom, R (eds) *Understanding Family Diversity and Home–School Relations* (pp 104–119). Abingdon: Routledge.

House of Commons (2016–17)
Children and Young People's Mental Health – the Role of Education: First Joint Report of the Education and Health Committees of Session 2016–17. London: House of Commons.

House of Commons (2018)
The Government's Green Paper on Mental Health: Failing a Generation. London: House of Commons Education and Health and Social Care Committees.

Jamal, F, Fletcher, A, Harden, A, Wells, H, Thomas, J and Bonell, C (2013)
The School Environment and Student Health: A Systematic Review and Meta-Ethnography of Qualitative Research. *BMC Public Health,* 13(798): 1–11.

Jeffcoat, T and Hayes, S C (2012)
A Randomized Trial of ACT Bibliotherapy on the Mental Health of K-12 Teachers and Staff. *Behaviour Research and Therapy,* 50(9): 571–9.

Johnston, D, Propper, C, Pudney, S and Shields M (2014)

Child Mental Health and Educational Attainment: Multiple Observers and the Measurement Error Problem. *Journal of Applied Economics*, 29: 880–900.

Klem, A M and Connell, J P (2004)

Relationships Matter: Linking Teacher Support to Student Engagement and Achievement. *Journal of School Health*, 74(7): 262–73.

Lave, J and Wenger, E (1991)

Situated Learning: Legitimate Peripheral Participation (Learning in Doing: Social, Cognitive and Computational Perspectives). Cambridge: Cambridge University Press.

Lilley, C, Ball, R and Vernon, H (2014)

The Experiences of 11–16 Year Olds on Social Networking Sites. London: NSPCC.

Lindsay, G and Dockrell, J (2012)

The Relationship Between Speech, Language and Communication Needs (SLCN) and Behavioural, Emotional and Social Difficulties. London: Department for Education.

Luthar S S (1993)

Annotation: Methodological and Conceptual Issues in the Study of Resilience. *Journal of Child Psychology and Psychiatry*, 34: 441–53.

McManus S, Bebbington P, Jenkins R and Brugha, T (2016)

Mental Health and Wellbeing in England: Adult Psychiatric Morbidity Survey 2014. Leeds: NHS digital.

Malecki, C K and Elliott, S N (2002)

Children's Social Behaviors as Predictors of Academic Achievement: A Longitudinal Analysis. *School Psychology Quarterly*, 17: 1–23.

Manning, V, Best, D W, Faulkner, N and Titherington, E (2009)

New Estimates of the Number of Children Living with Substance Misusing Parents: Results from UK National Household Surveys. *BMC Public Health*, 9(377): 1–12.

Masten, A S (2001)

Ordinary Magic: Resilience Processes in Development. *American Psychologist*, 56(3): 227–38.

National Institute for Health and Care Excellence (NICE) (2013)

Social and Emotional Wellbeing for Children and Young People. London: NICE.

Noble, C and Toft, M (2010)

Reducing Disaffection and Increasing School Engagement, in Aggleton, P, Dennison, C and Warwick, I (eds) *Promoting Health and Well-Being Through Schools* (pp 42–55). Abingdon: Routledge.

OECD (2016)

PISA 2015 Results, *Students' Wellbeing Volume III*. OECD, April 2016. [online] Available at: www.oecd.org/edu/pisa-2015-results-volume-iii-9789264273856-en.htm (accessed 15 July 2018).

Office for National Statistics (ONS) (2015)

Measuring National Well-being: Insights into Children's Mental Health and Well-being. [online] Available at: www.ons.gov.uk/peoplepopulation andcommunity/wellbeing/articles/measuringnationalwellbeing/2015-10-20 (accessed 8 August 2018).

Office for National Statistics (ONS) (2016)

Internet Access – Households and Individuals: 2016. [online] Available at: www. ons.gov.uk/peoplepopulationandcommunity/householdcharacteristics/homeintern etandsocialmediausage/bulletins/internetaccesshouseholdsandindividuals/2016 (accessed 8 August 2018).

O'Hara, M (2014)

Teachers Left to Pick up Pieces from Cuts to Youth Mental Health Services. [online] Available at: www.theguardian.com/education/2014/apr/15/pupils-mental-health-cuts-services-stress-teachers (accessed 8 August 2018).

Patel, V, Flisher, A J, Nikapota, A and Malhotra, S (2008)

Promoting Child and Adolescent Mental Health in Low and Middle Income Countries. *Journal of Child Psychology and Psychiatry*, 49: 313–14.

Paterson, A and Grantham, R (2016)

How to Make Teachers Happy: An Exploration of Teacher Wellbeing in the Primary School Context. *Journal of Educational & Child Psychology*, 33(2): 90–104.

Payne, E and Smith, M (2013)

LGBTQ Kids, School Safety, and Missing the Big Picture: How the Dominant Bullying Discourse Prevents School Professionals from Thinking about Systemic Marginalization or ... Why We Need to Rethink LGBTQ Bullying. *QED*, 1(1): 1–36.

Prever, M (2006)

Mental Health in Schools. London: Paul Chapman.

Pryzbylski, A, Murayama, K, DeHaan, C and Gladwell, V (2013)

Motivational, Emotional and Behavioural Correlates of Fear of Missing Out. *Computers in Human Behaviour*, 29(4): 1841–8.

Public Health England (PHE) (2015)
Promoting Children and Young People's Emotional Health and Wellbeing: A Whole School and College Approach. London: PHE.

Roffey, S (2012)
Pupil Wellbeing–Teacher Wellbeing: Two Sides of the Same Coin? *Educational and Child Psychology*, 29(4): 8–17.

Roffey, S (2017)
Ordinary Magic Needs Ordinary Magicians: The Power and Practice of Positive Relationships for Building Youth Resilience and Wellbeing. *Kognition und Paedagogik*, 103: 38–57.

Royal Society for Public Health (RSPH) (2017)
#StatusOfMind: Social Media and Young People's Mental Health and Wellbeing. London: RSPH.

Sammons, P (2007)
A Review of School Effectiveness and Improvement. [online] Available at: www.cfbt.com/evidenceforeducation/pdf/Full%20Literature%20Review.pdf (accessed 8 August 2018).

Scott, H, Gardani, M, Biello, S and Woods, H (2016)
Social Media Use, Fear of Missing Out and Sleep Outcomes in Adolescents. [online] Available at: www.researchgate.net/publication/308903222_Social_media_use_fear_of_missing_out_and_sleep_outcomes_in_adolescence (accessed 8 August 2018).

Sidebotham, P, Brandon, M, Bailey, S, Belderson, P, Dodsworth, J, Garstang, J, Harrison, E, Retzer, A and Sorensen, P (2016)
Pathways to Harm, Pathways to Protection: A Triennial Analysis of Serious Case Reviews 2011 to 2014. London: DfE.

Sisak, M, Varnick, P, Varnik, A, Apter, A, Balazs, J, Balint, M and Wasserman, D (2014)
Teacher Satisfaction with School and Psychological Well-Being Affects Readiness to Help Children with Mental Health Problems. *Health Education Journal*, 73: 382–93.

Spenrath, M A, Clarke, M E and Kutcher, S (2011)
The Science of Brain and Biological Development: Implications for Mental Health Research, Practice and Policy. *Journal of the Canadian Academy of Child and Adolescent Psychiatry*, 20(4): 298–304.

Stewart-Brown, S (2006)

What is the Evidence on School Health Promotion in Improving Health or Preventing Disease and, Specifically, What is the Effectiveness of the Health Promoting Schools Approach? Copenhagen: WHO Regional Office for Europe.

Strathie, S, Strathie, C and Kennedy, H (2011)

Video Enhanced Reflective Practice (VERP), in Kennedy, H, Landor, M and Todd, L (eds) *Video Interaction Guidance: A Relationship-Based Intervention to Promote Attunement, Empathy and Wellbeing* (pp 170–80). London: Jessica Kingsley.

Teo, A, Carlson, E, Mathieu, P J, Egeland, B and Sroufe, L A (1996)

A Prospective Longitudinal Study of Psychosocial Predictors of Academic Achievement. *Journal of School Psychology*, 34: 285–306.

Thapa, A, Cohen, J Guffey, S and Alessandro, A (2013)

A Review of School Climate Research. *Review of Educational Research,* 83(3): 357–85.

Tiggemann, M and Slater, A E (2013)

NetGirls: The Internet, Facebook and Body Image Concern in Adolescent Girls. *International Journal of Eating Disorders*, 46(6): 630–3.

Tiggemann, M and Slater A E (2014)

NetTweens: The Internet and Body Image Concerns in Preteenage Girls. *Journal of Early Adolescence*, 34(5): 606–20.

Time to Change (2015)

Campaign Set to Tackle Life-Limiting Mental Health Stigma Among Teens. [online] Available at: www.time-to-change.org.uk/news/new-campaign-set-tackle-life-limiting-mental-health-stigma-among-teens (accessed 8 August 2018).

Watson, T (2014)

Teachers' Wellbeing: Under Scrutiny and Under-Appreciated. [online] Available at: www.theguardian.com/teacher-network/teacher-blog/2014/jul/01/teachers-wellbeing-under-scrutiny-underappreciated (accessed 8 August 2018).

Weare, K (2010)

Promoting Mental Health Through Schools, in Aggleton, P, Dennison, C and Warwick, I (eds) *Promoting Health and Well-being Through Schools* (pp 24–41). Abingdon: Routledge.

Weare, K and Markham, W (2005)

What Do We Know About Promoting Mental Health Through Schools? *Promotion and Education*, 12: 118–22.

Welsh, M, Parke, R D, Widaman, K and O'Neil, R (2001)

Linkages Between Children's Social and Academic Competence: A Longitudinal Analysis. *Journal of School Psychology*, 39: 463–82.

Wentzel, K R (1993)

Does Being Good Make the Grade? Social Behavior and Academic Competence in Middle School. *Journal of Educational Psychology*, 85: 357–64.

Wood, J J (2006)

Effect of Anxiety Reduction on Children's School Performance and Adjustment. *Developmental Psychology*, 42: 345–9.

Woods, H C and Scott, H (2016)

#Sleepyteens: Social Media Use in Adolescence is Associated with Poor Sleep Quality, Anxiety, Depression and Low Self-esteem. *Journal of Adolescence*, 51: 41–9.

World Health Organisation (WHO) (2014)

Mental Health: A State of Wellbeing. [online] www.who.int/features/factfiles/mental_health/en (accessed 3 August 2018).

Xanidid, N and Brignell, C (2016)

The Association Between the Use of Social Network Sites, Sleep and Cognitive Function During the Day. *Computers in Human Behaviour*, 55: 121–6.

Zins, J E, Bloodworth, M R, Weissberg, R P and Walberg, H J (2004)

The Scientific Base Linking Social and Emotional Learning to School Success, in Zins, J, Weissberg, R, Wang, M and Walberg, H J (eds) *Building Academic Success on Social and Emotional Learning: What Does the Research Say?* (pp 3–22). New York: Teachers College Press.

+INDEX